**D**

- The number one reason for decreased sexual desire?
- Which herbs increase a woman's sexual energy?
- The ancient Taoist secrets of oral sex?
- The foods that work as natural aphrodisiacs?
- The techniques of "The Valley Orgasm" for achieving the peak of sexual pleasure?
- The ways erotica, role playing, and fantasies can turn your love life into a sexual adventure?

Discover the answers to these questions and many more in this authoritative guide to . . .

# *Natural Sex*

**Elena Oumano,** Ph.D., teaches at the City University of New York. She specializes in the fields of natural Western and Eastern healing arts, and is an expert in such techniques as herbology, yoga, acupressure, massage, and homeopathy. She has written articles for many national magazines and newspapers, including the *New York Times, Los Angeles Times, Village Voice,* and *Newsday,* and is the author of several books on relationships and natural healing. She lives in New York City.

# *Natural Sex*

ELENA OUMANO, PH.D.

A LYNN SONBERG BOOK

A PLUME BOOK

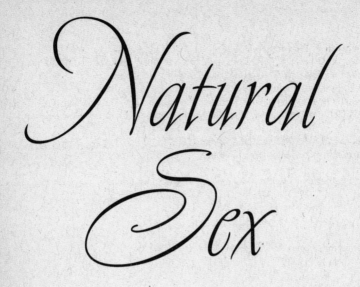

PLUME
Published by the Penguin Group
Penguin Putnam Inc., 375 Hudson Street, New York, New York 10014, U.S.A.
Penguin Books Ltd, 27 Wrights Lane, London W8 5TZ, England
Penguin Books Australia Ltd, Ringwood, Victoria, Australia
Penguin Books Canada Ltd, 10 Alcorn Avenue, Toronto, Ontario, Canada M4V 3B2
Penguin Books (N.Z.) Ltd, 182–190 Wairau Road, Auckland 10, New Zealand

Penguin Books Ltd, Registered Offices:
Harmondsworth, Middlesex, England

First published by Plume, a member of Penguin Putnam Inc.

First Printing, February, 1999
10 9 8 7 6 5 4 3 2 1



LIBRARY OF CONGRESS CATALOGING-IN-PUBLICATION DATA

Oumano, Elena.
Natural sex / Elena Oumano.
p. cm.
ISBN 0-452-28048-6
1. Sex. 2. Sexual disorders—Diet therapy. I. Title.
HQ23.092 1999
306.7—dc21 98-42311
CIP

Printed in the United States of America
Set in Bitstream Charter
Designed by Stanley S. Drate / Folio Graphics Co. Inc.

# Acknowledgments

I am grateful to Lynn Sonberg for her invaluable conceptual and editorial input. Many thanks to my literary agent, Madeleine Morel, for her consistently helpful guidance and for listening. The chapter on herbs and supplements benefited substantially from the input of David I. F. Miller, biochemist and nutritional consultant. And thanks to my editors, Deirdre Mullane and Jennifer Dickerson—this book would not have been possible without your dedication, enthusiasm, and keen insights. Last, my thanks go to the men and women whose experience forms the backbone of this book.

# Contents

## *Part Two*

## GREAT SEX, NATURALLY

# Preface

It is my experience that the preservation of sexual vitality is a primary concern of many people. Consider the enormous sums of money spent each year on enhancing physical appearances, or the past excitement and publicity surrounding news of the sex drug Viagra. Clearly, our society has an overwhelming need to reclaim our sexual satisfaction.

But the question remains: how do we safeguard our sexual health and address the daunting problem of sexual dysfunction? Providing answers is the goal of Elena Oumano's book, *Natural Sex,* and no one else has done so as thoroughly or as cogently.

This book presents the most comprehensive and effective approaches to enhancing sexual function that I have ever encountered. Rather than treating sexual problems as isolated phenomena, Oumano views them as reflections of underlying health issues. Accordingly, her advice is geared toward improving general health first by making dietary and other lifestyle changes, then by specifically addressing sexual function. Even more pertinent, Oumano takes a holistic view of health and sexuality. All the remedies, exercises, and other techniques and strategies she recommends are natural. That is, they carry little or no side effects and benefit one's entire being—body, mind, and sexual function.

*Natural Sex* is actually a comprehensive guide to sexual self-healing the natural way. Among the many topics Oumano covers are herbs and supplements that protect and enhance sexual function, as well as extensive and detailed discussions and explanations of yoga techniques, taoist exercises, body-mind exercises to release emotional blocks, and various relaxation exercises. She even includes valuable information on how imagination and color visualization can enhance sexual pleasure. The sections on sexual techniques are equally far-ranging and informative, including role playing, fantasies, and Eastern lovemaking practices. The discussion on orgasm is perceptive, honest, and eminently helpful.

The book concludes with a chapter that delivers sound information on proven aphrodisiacs and a final chapter that tells how natural remedies and techniques can preserve one's sexual vitality in the later years of life, covering the gamut from traditional wisdom to the latest cutting-edge discoveries.

In short, anyone can benefit from the sage counsel and detailed information presented in *Natural Sex.* Readers not only can expect improvement in the quality of their sex lives, but better general health and increased energy. The holistic and natural approach taken by *Natural Sex* is far superior to any of the quick-fix solutions—the drugs, prosthetics, and surgical techniques—that are so widely publicized in our media.

—ERIC S. ROTH, M.D., board-certified in physical medicine and rehabilitation, and graduate of the New York College of Osteopathic Medicine's accelerated program for medical doctors

# Introduction

Most of us long for a truly impassioned sex life. But no matter what our current level of satisfaction, whether we regularly reach Nirvana or find ourselves on the outside looking in, most of us would like to increase our erotic pleasure.

The truth is that for many of us, sexual satisfaction is an elusive mystery. It's on the movie screen, it's in books, it certainly occupies our imaginations, but somehow it isn't in our bedrooms.

Many of us are frustrated, or at least bothered by the feeling that something is amiss. We lack the sexual energy that inspires us to initiate and respond to the moment. We do not achieve the deep orgasmic pleasure we crave and settle instead for sexual sensations that, while pleasurable, lack intensity and fervor. And far too many of us are plagued by chronic, common sex-related problems that can make it hard to enjoy any physical intimacy at all.

We don't know what's wrong, but it is clear that whatever we've done to date is not enough.

Psychotherapists have helped uncover deep-seated psychological causes for sexual inhibitions, fears, and dysfunctions. Sex therapists have helped break down intimacy barriers and offered techniques for sensual touching so that people can come to know themselves and their lovers better and more fully.

Yet many of us are still experiencing all manner of blocks that affect our sexual vitality, health, and pleasure.

This book is the outcome of my many years studying myriad natural alternative treatments that focus on the person as a holistic entity—as a physical, mental, spiritual, and sexual being. It also brings together the results of my explorations into the interrelationship between sexual satisfaction and health, a connection too often ignored by sex researchers and manuals, which tend to compartmentalize sex, treating it as separate and distinct from the other aspects of our experience. This book's aim is to correct that prevalent viewpoint, as well as to reveal how both traditional Eastern disciplines and cutting-edge alternative Western healing systems can be used to achieve passionate, happy sex lives.

*Natural Sex* draws together the best of these Eastern and Western philosophies, remedies, and techniques into an easy-to-use format, to help anyone overcome sexual blocks and enjoy greater sexual pleasure and satisfaction.

This book also focuses on developing good health along with sexual fulfillment. A full, satisfying sex life is greatly enhanced by the high level of vitality that results from good health. The components of good health are exercise, proper diet, adequate rest, preventative medicine, and psychological, spiritual, and sexual well-being.

Just as health affects our sexuality, sexuality affects our health. Sex not only feels good; it's good for you. Enjoying sexual intimacy with another person enables excellent health to permeate your entire being because sex actually nourishes you. According to many research studies, lovemaking and orgasm boost circulation, improve skin tone, strengthen the immune system, release tension, and promote psychological health. Sex has been shown to relieve the minor pain of headaches and arthritis and other complaints, possibly because the brain releases endorphins, the body's natural painkillers, during orgasm. In women, regular sex can prevent unwelcome changes to the vagina that accompany menopause, such as dryness and slackened muscle tone. Some studies even indicate that sex is good for your heart.

So sexual desire and fulfillment are linked to physical, emotional, and spiritual health in ways far deeper than most of us imagine. And sexual problems cannot be isolated from your overall health.

The number one complaint made by both men and women is lack of sexual desire. For women, the second most common sexual problem is the inability to reach orgasm during intercourse. The issue of female orgasm is still clouded by misinformation and the heated debate over which type of orgasm is better, clitoral or vaginal. The sad truth is, for too many women any kind of orgasm is an elusive pleasure. Most studies report that between 10 and 15 percent of women never climax, even during masturbation. Another 20 to 30 percent do so only by masturbation. Approximately the same percentage have never climaxed during intercourse. Finally, a tiny percentage of women may experience something called a "missed orgasm." They exhibit the physiological signs, including vaginal contractions, but they don't feel the climax, probably because they are denying themselves that pleasure for various psychological reasons.

But with all the concern over women's orgasms, the subject of male orgasm has gone sadly neglected. One of the best kept sexual secrets is that ejaculation does not necessarily mean that a man's been sexually satisfied, that he's experienced a full body orgasm.

Whether the problem is male or female orgasm or a host of other common sexual complaints and insecurities about our bodies, most can be resolved easily through good nutrition, various supplements, exercises, techniques, guided visualizations, and other natural remedies described in this book. In fact, these practices often work better than Western medicine's pharmaceuticals and surgical interventions, which bring with them potentially harmful side effects.

In short, you don't need whipped cream, camcorders, bizarre lovemaking apparatus, or years of costly psychotherapy to have a great sex life. All you need is the right information.

Once you understand the deep interconnection of overall health to optimum sexuality, any sexual dysfunction becomes merely a feedback message that you can deal with and resolve.

You'll realize that your body knows how to heal itself, after you remove any stressors or misunderstandings. Sexual fulfillment will become an overall restorative for you and your partner, even a system of mutual healing and awakening of the spirit.

Why do we need to turn to the wisdom of the East for sexual guidance? In part, because Western sex is so goal oriented, so based on the rigid mechanics of tension and release.

Eastern sex is about letting go and giving yourself up to the *experience.* While orgasm is the crowning pleasure of most sexual encounters, many people never reach this climax because they are tense, performance oriented, or trying too hard. Traditional Western advice tends toward a "Let's Fix It" agenda, as if sexuality were a machine and all people have to do is become mechanical masters. Just a little tinkering with the parts, and we'll be motoring off to orgasm. To experience the most pleasurable sexual sensations, we need to open ourselves to the many available natural solutions.

This book describes a wide variety of time-tested natural healing and medicinal systems. It supplies nutritional, herbal, and supplemental remedies that support, tone, and prepare the body for deeper, more intense lovemaking. It tells you how proven aphrodisiacs, body-mind techniques, massage, acupuncture, ancient Chinese and Indian sex exercises and lovemaking techniques, as well as innovative modern Western practices that spring from traditional Eastern practices will increase your sexual vitality, pleasure, health, and satisfaction. This is the only book that shows you how the pool of practical information offered by the East and holistic West can enhance your sexual health, excitement, and orgasm. This wisdom will provide you with remedies and practices that improve sexual energy, endurance, and pleasure and, at the same time, prevent common sex problems that can keep you from enjoying sex fully. Those problems can range from long-term sex-related complaints—such as impotence, premature ejaculation, or lack of orgasmic experience—that require consistent use of a remedy or technique, to problems that can be resolved by quick solutions.

In short, this book addresses every aspect of your sexuality. It explores with absolute frankness the empty, dull, uncomfortable, even painful moments in our sex lives and offers natural choices and solutions. Understanding our own bodies as well as those of our lovers can be a joyful process. We need to "let go" and experience ourselves as sexual beings.

Sexuality is a core aspect of your humanity that requires recognition, nurturance, even your emotional and spiritual attention. This book wants to inspire that vision in you.

# Part One

## SEXUAL VITALITY: PREPARING MIND AND BODY FOR GREAT SEX

# 1

# THE FOOD CONNECTION

Soybeans instead of estrogen supplements? Fenugreek seeds to cure impotency? That's right! Smart food choices can help give you the supercharged sex life you've always wanted. Far from being an isolated act, sex is a holistic activity that involves the health of your entire being—body, mind, and soul.

Crucial dietary chemicals in food protect and boost your overall health and vitality, which in turn prevent and heal disturbances in your sexual function. On the other hand, an unhealthy diet robs your body of the nutrients it needs for a strong libido and passionate lovemaking.

Work pressures, emotional problems, stress, medications, allergies, and other factors can also play havoc with your sex life. But when you look beyond all these components, more often than not, you will discover the underlying cause is a long-term poor diet. Inadequate nutrition weakens the entire body—brain, nerves, genitals, endocrine glands, heart, blood vessels, and other organs—leaving you without the energy and stamina needed to fulfill your erotic potential.

Health-care providers report that the number one health complaint today is lack of energy. Not surprisingly, the number one *sexual* complaint is lack of sufficient energy to enjoy sex. Many people are simply too tired to become fully aroused and engage in passionate lovemaking. You don't have to be sick to be sluggish and disinterested in sex. Depleting the body of health and vitality through unhealthy eating habits lays the foundation for eventual disease and dysfunction—especially of the sex organs and glands.

People fuel their fast-paced, pressure-filled modern lives with fast foods: soft drinks chock-full of sugar or artificial sweeteners, cups of coffee, saturated fats, quick-fix simple carbohydrates, and chemical additives. While these can provide a quick burst of energy, they offer little nutrition beyond that short-lived jolt. And, as we all know, what goes up will come down.

Eating the wrong foods erodes not only your overall physical vitality. It saps your sexual health. If you are young, you probably don't feel the effects of your substandard diet. Ten, twenty, or thirty years down the road, though, that inadequate nutritional investment will leave you sexually short-changed. Your only dividends will be deteriorated health, chronic fatigue, and a lackluster or even nonexistent sex life.

The good news is that you determine the quality of your health. It's under your control. Eat right and you will experience a greater degree of sexual desire, enhance your ability to perform, and achieve more frequent, intense orgasms. Good nutrition is not just your best sex booster; it protects your long-term sexual health and helps you enjoy a lifetime of passionate lovemaking. Simply follow the advice in this chapter and you will be taking an important step toward overcoming that far too common "too tired for sex" syndrome.

Let's take a look at the overall health picture to see how your body functions best. All foods are made up of proteins, fats, and carbohydrates in various proportions. The key to good nutrition, and good sex, is to choose those food sources that supply these basic elements in the right quantities. People who live in cultures where the diet includes fresh fruits, vegetables, nuts, seeds, and grains and less hydrogenated fats have far less incidence of heart and circulation disease. They also experience much fewer sexual problems and infertility.

U.S. government nutritionists recommend that your daily diet be composed of 40 percent carbohydrates, 30 percent protein, and 30 percent fats—a plan commonly known as the "food pyramid." Although some experts in the natural medicine field dispute those percentages, one point on which most experts agree is a person's daily fat intake should be 30 percent or less of the daily caloric intake. One of these, the American Heart Association, recommends a diet rich in grains, fruits, and vegetables and advises that heart-harmful saturated fats be held at just 10 percent.

What does this mean in terms of optimal sexual health? Just that we are what we eat. So let's take a look at some of the major building blocks of what, exactly, we are.

## SEX VITAMINS AND MINERALS

You need a full range of vitamins and minerals—essential body chemicals—to protect your overall health and stimulate a hearty sexual appetite. Certain body chemicals are particularly important to your love life.

Some people mistakenly believe they can eat substandard foods and make up for it by popping vitamin and mineral pills. But it's always best to get daily nutrients in their natural, whole form. Unfortunately, in this era of modern industrial mega-farms, overprocessed foods, and chemical pollution, it's not always possible to get all the vitamins and minerals needed through food—no matter how much you are trying to make the right dietary choices. Many foods *look* fresh and healthy, but are actually low in the nutrients they would have if they had been grown and/or raised under natural conditions.

Use the following list of vitamins and minerals and their food sources to guide your daily dietary choices and to ensure that you are getting as much nutrition as possible from your food. Chapter 3 will give you additional information on how supplements can help you meet your daily nutritional quota and protect your sexual health.

### VITAMINS

#### *Vitamin E*

Popularly known as "the sex vitamin," vitamin E plays a key role in other areas as well. When you become sexually excited, oxygen-bearing blood floods your sex organs, causing them to swell, and become erect and more sensitive. Vitamin E helps the blood transport energizing oxygen to your sex organs. At the same time it ensures the oxygen won't cause those tissues to oxidize. It is an extremely effective antioxidant, which means that it prevents your body's cells from merging with oxygen, which then destroys them. Many researchers believe that antioxidants like vitamin E are a key part of cancer prevention.

Vitamin E also helps postmenopausal women and women who have undergone hysterectomies make up for the loss of estrogen. It eases related symptoms such as hot flashes; dry, thinning vaginal tissue; and loss of libido. In addition, E boosts fertility in women of childbearing age.

Another reason to maintain strong vitamin E levels is its benefit to the pituitary gland, known as the body's "master gland," in part because of its influence on sex organ function and sexual characteristics. Some holistic healers prescribe extra doses of E to relieve general vaginitis (inflammation and irritation of the vaginal tissue) and to prevent prostatitis (inflammation of the male prostate gland).

It's difficult to get the levels of vitamin E you need from food alone, especially if you're over forty, when your supply of this vitamin starts to lower and your need increases. See chapter 3 for guidelines on supplementing this essential nutrient.

*NUTRITIONAL SOURCES OF E:* Vitamin E is found mostly in unrefined grain products such as wheat, rye, oats, corn, as well as bran and wheat germ. It is also found in abundance in soybeans, peanuts, asparagus, salmon, butter, spinach, nuts, sunflower seeds, and in oils made from sunflower seeds, safflower seeds, almonds, sesame seeds, peanuts, corn, wheat germ, olives, and soybeans.

### *Vitamin A*

Vitamin A is needed to maintain sex hormone function in both men and women and is especially essential for healthy testicular tissue and adequate sperm levels. There are two types of vitamin A: retinol, which comes from animal sources, and carotenoids, which are derived from vegetables and fruits and are converted by the body into vitamin A.

Commercial processing robs food of vitamin A, usually by boiling it out. On the other hand, this fat-soluble vitamin is stored in the liver, so taking too much vitamin A in supplements can be toxic. Fortunately, fresh vegetables are a wonderful source, so eat your veggies.

*NUTRITIONAL SOURCES OF A:* Vegetables: carrots, sweet potatoes, sweet peppers, red chili peppers, pumpkin, yams, yellow zucchini, winter squash, hubbard squash, acorn squash, dark leafy greens (collard greens, kale, spinach, endive, cabbage, beet greens, watercress, romaine lettuce, swiss chard, turnip greens), chives, parsley, broccoli, corn and corn products, and green onions.

Fruits: apricots (especially dried), peaches, nectarines, cantaloupe, papaya, mango, and prunes.

Animal products: liver, fish (especially white fish and shellfish), and dairy products (especially yellow butter and cream).

Eggs: Despite the bad rap eggs have received because of their high cholesterol content, raw eggs contain lecithin, which acts as an antidote to dietary cholesterol. If you are certain that your supply of raw eggs is safe (check with your health-food store), eat raw eggs to give yourself a wonderful and dense source of many nutrients, including vitamin A. You can blend one or two raw eggs with a natural fruit juice for an energizing morning drink.

### *Vitamin C*

Vitamin C has been proven to help prevent miscarriages, and mounting evidence suggests that this water-soluble vitamin can also help you enjoy more explosive, longer-lasting orgasms and keep the skin soft and supple. As you age, your sex glands need more and more vitamin C. If your levels are low, your sex life will suffer.

*NUTRITIONAL SOURCES OF C:* Virtually all vegetables and fruits contain vitamin C, but the following vegetables and fruits are particularly rich in this important nutrient.

Vegetables: leafy greens (kale, collard greens, turnip greens, swiss chard, mustard greens, watercress, spinach, cabbage), all sprouts, sweet peppers, red chili peppers, parsley, brussels sprouts, broccoli, okra, lima beans, blackeyed peas, soybeans, green peas, cauliflower, asparagus, green onions, the skin of baked or boiled potatoes.

Fruits: citrus fruits (orange, grapefruit, lemon, lime), dried fruits, fruit juices and fruit sauces, all berries (especially strawberries).

Animal products: Liver, oysters.

### *Bioflavonoids*

Bioflavonoids work in your body in tandem with vitamin C and are often found together in foods, particularly in the white pulp under the skin of citrus fruits. That is why it's best to eat the whole fruit rather than just the juice, so you can reap the benefits of this nutritional synergy.

Among other fruits and vegetables that contain bioflavonoids are grapes, rose hips, prunes, cherries, black currants, plums, apricots, blackberries, papaya, cantaloupe, tomatoes, parsley, peppers, cabbage, and broccoli.

### *B Complex*

The B vitamins are known as the energy vitamins, and they are essential for a healthy, balanced nervous system. Without energy and a strong nervous system, your sexual apparatus cannot function properly. The Bs also boost levels of testosterone, the male sex hormone that is also present in females—although in far lower levels—and is responsible for "turning on" both sexes. Consuming adequate amounts of all the Bs is important, because they work together. So eat from a variety of vitamin B–rich foods to perk up your libido and keep your sex machinery running smoothly.

Vitamin $B_1$ (also known as thiamine) helps maintain your thyroid gland. If you're low in $B_1$, you risk developing an underactive thyroid, which will put a damper on sexual desire and function.

$B_2$ (aka riboflavin), $B_3$ (aka niacin), and another B vitamin called pantothenic acid tone and strengthen your adrenal glands. In traditional Eastern medicine the adrenals (which sit atop the kidneys) are thought to control sexual function, as well as your general energy levels and resistance to disease. Even conventional Western doctors know that if adrenal function is low, sexual desire and performance suffer.

Folic acid, another B, works with testosterone to produce

sperm. It also protects the response of the reproductive organs to estrogen. Low levels can also worsen menopausal symptoms. $B_{12}$ is used to treat male sterility and female infertility, and to fuel energy. Para-aminobenzoic acid (aka PABA) is used to maintain healthy penile tissue, especially in older men.

*NUTRITIONAL SOURCES OF VITAMIN B:* All whole grain foods contain high levels of B complex vitamins. Eat them instead of refined starches. Other foods high in the Bs include peanuts, nuts, seeds, legumes, pork, leafy greens (especially collard greens, kale, parsley, cabbage, and spinach), broccoli, mushrooms, hot red peppers, potatoes, milk and milk products (especially aged cheese), brewer's yeast, lamb kidneys, lamb, chicken liver, chicken, egg yolk, lobster, mackerel, salmon, trout, halibut, perch, tuna, clams, oysters, turkey, royal jelly (made from bees), raisins, cantaloupe, bananas, avocado, molasses, flaxseed, apricots, apples, cherries, peaches, plums, and nectarines.

## MINERALS

While many foods boost your sex drive and function, those containing high amounts of minerals are near the top of the list. In general, good sources of minerals are found in mineral water and root vegetables like onions, potatoes, carrots, turnips, and yams.

### *Calcium, Magnesium, and Phosphorus*

We group these three minerals because they work together in the body. Many people are aware that the calcium-to-magnesium ratio should be approximately two to one. Fewer realize that the phosphorus-calcium-magnesium ratio is also important for optimum health, particularly of the sex organs and glands. Your body needs substantial amounts of phosphorus, and it must work in a specific ratio with calcium, particularly to prevent menopausal symptoms. Here's the equation: for every 1,000 mg of calcium, you need 500 mg of magnesium and 400 mg of phosphorus. If you are over forty or are allergic to dairy products, you need to take calcium-magnesium or calcium-magnesium-phosphorus supplements that conform to the standard ratio of these three essential minerals.

*NUTRITIONAL SOURCES OF CALCIUM:* Foods high in calcium include milk and milk products, uncooked vegetables (especially dark, leafy vegetables like kale, collard greens, mustard greens, beet greens, turnip greens, dandelion greens, watercress, spinach, lettuce, as well as parsley, cabbage, brussels sprouts, and broccoli), sesame seeds, sunflower seeds, whole oats, dried beans (navy beans, soybeans), sardines, salmon, almonds, walnuts, peanuts, brazil nuts, kelp, dulse, carob, dried figs, sunflower seeds, wheat bran, raw buckwheat, ripe olives.

*NUTRITIONAL SOURCES OF MAGNESIUM:* Foods high in magnesium include kelp, wheat bran, wheat germ, almonds, cashews, blackstrap molasses, buckwheat, brazil nuts, dulse, filberts, peanuts, millet, wheat grain, pecans, English walnuts, rye, beet greens, coconut meat, soybeans, spinach, brown rice, dried figs, swiss chard, apricots, dates.

*NUTRITIONAL SOURCES OF PHOSPHORUS:* Among the foods rich in phosphorus are truffles, egg yolk (lecithin), fish, wheat bran, pumpkin seeds, squash seeds, sunflower seeds, sesame seeds, brazil nuts, almonds, walnuts, cashews, peanuts, pinto beans, rye, millet, dulse, kelp, chicken, crab, beef, lamb, lentils, mushrooms, garlic, sweet corn, raisins, yogurt, and brussels sprouts.

### *Zinc*

Zinc is particularly essential for production of the male hormone testosterone. As we age, our zinc levels decline. If you smoke, drink alcohol, and/or coffee, or suffer from infections, you are also losing zinc and putting yourself at risk for low testosterone levels. This will cause lowered libido, impotency, and overall weak sexual functioning in both sexes. Increasingly, natural health-care providers are blaming low zinc levels for inflammation and swelling of the prostate gland (prostatitis), a near-epidemic condition affecting men over fifty, and for insufficient vaginal lubrication in mature women. Low zinc levels are also thought to cause low sperm count and poor development of the penis and testes. While zinc supplements are often prescribed, your best bet is to protect yourself with dietary sources of zinc.

*NUTRITIONAL SOURCES OF ZINC:* Foods that contain high levels of zinc include oysters (considered an aphrodisiac because they contain the most zinc of any food), raw eggs, green peas, split peas, lentils, pecans, brazil nuts, hazel nuts (filberts), peanuts, lima beans, soy lecithin, almonds, walnuts, sardines, chicken, buckwheat, ginger root, whole wheat, oats, rye, beef, beef liver, lamb, clams, anchovies, tuna, haddock.

### *Iron*

Iron is necessary for the manufacture of hemoglobin, which transports oxygen to your body's tissues, including your sex organs and glands. If your iron levels are low, your tissues become oxygen-starved due to insufficient red blood cells, and your energy plummets.

*NUTRITIONAL SOURCES OF IRON:* Foods containing high amounts of iron include apricots, peaches, bananas, black molasses, dates, prunes, raisins, brewer's yeast, whole grains and whole grain products, farina, turnip greens, broccoli, brussels sprouts, spinach, beet greens, alfalfa, beets, asparagus, sunflower seeds, sesame seeds, walnuts and other nuts, dry beans, lentils, kelp, egg yolk, red meat, beef, all organ meats, raw clams, oysters, coffee, chocolate.

### *Serotonin*

Some experts blame low serotonin levels for insufficient ejaculations and low sperm count. This sex chemical is produced by the brain from carbohydrates that combine with foods containing the amino acid tryptophane, which is found in turkey and other meats, as well as in dairy products. Serotonin can also be lost through excess stress. Try such combinations as fish, poultry, or lean beef with bread, whole grains, or pasta.

## Nature's Sex Foods

Cultivate the health and vitality you need for a more passionate love life by eating a wide variety of the nutrient-rich foods listed below.

*FRUITS:* apples, bananas, plums, pineapple, cherries, pears, raisins, grapes, avocado, pomegranates, quinces, melons, figs, dates, apricots, peaches, nectarines, oranges, grapefruits, lemons, limes.

*VEGETABLES:* Beets, radishes, onions, garlic, cucumber, celery, artichokes, green beans, peas, asparagus, okra, mushrooms, parsnip, corn, eggplant, broccoli, cauliflower sprouts, all green leafy vegetables.

*WHOLE GRAINS:* Wheat, rice, millet, oats, barley, rye, buckwheat, cornmeal, bulgur, triticale.

*LEGUMES:* Lentils, peanuts, dried peas, dried beans, soy, mung, black kidney, red kidney, chick pea (garbanzo), pinto, lima, aduki, great northern, black-eyed peas, navy, white.

*NUTS AND SEEDS:* Almonds, cashews, brazil nuts, walnuts, filberts (hazel nuts), pine nuts, nut butters, sunflower, pumpkin, sesame, fenugreek, squash seeds, and their seed butters, such as tahini (made from sesame seeds). Note: You don't need to consume tremendous portions of these foods. Small but frequent servings are best, as nuts and seeds pack a lot of nutrition and their caloric and fat contents are also sky-high!

*ANIMAL PROTEINS:* Eggs, fish, poultry (remove the skin before eating), lean red meat.

### *Plant Versus Animal Proteins*

Many advocates of vegetarianism suggest combining whole grains, like brown rice, with legumes, like soybeans, to make a complete protein meal. But these combinations are not exactly complete: they lack certain key enzymes and do not deliver vitamin $B_{12}$ in a form that your body can metabolize easily.

On the other hand, too much protein—particularly animal protein—can deliver excessive quantities of saturated fat and tax your liver, impairing its metabolism of sugars and possibly leading to hypoglycemia and chronic fatigue. We do need animal protein in our diets, but animal protein intake should not be excessive. To maintain an optimum sexual response, men should limit animal protein intake to four to six ounces per day, while women do not need to eat more than three to five ounces of meat a day.

If you are a woman who needs to increase and/or balance her estrogen levels, snack on soybean products and substitute them for animal protein at least one meal a day. Among the soy products you can use are tofu, soy flour, soy milk, soy cheese, and soy grits. To create almost complete plant proteins, try these tasty grain-legume-nut combinations:

rice and beans
millet and peas
whole grain bread with tofu spread
baked beans and whole grain bread
millet pudding
millet croquettes
low-fat granola and/or nuts and seeds
lentil soup with sunflower seeds
bean, grain, and nut casserole
soy milk custard with chopped nuts
bean spread and whole grain bread
rice and sesame seeds
seed butter spread on whole grain bread
bulgur and bean salad

See the appendix for recommended vegetarian cookbooks.

## Nature's Sex Diet

The following sample meals give you an idea of the kinds of food combinations that provide the quality nutrition your body needs to protect your long-term health and youthful vitality, build a healthy sexual appetite, and enjoy the kind of sexual fireworks that lift your spirits like nothing else.

### BREAKFAST

Some people prefer to start the day with a glass of juice. A far better idea is to eat the whole fruit so that you get all its nutrients in balanced form. If you are hypoglycemic and/or suffer from recurrent yeast infections, eat a fruit that's low in sugar, like grapefruit or papaya, or skip fruit altogether. Try something like this:

Orange (vitamin C), banana (riboflavin), or papaya (vitamin A and digestive enzymes)

Whole grain cereal with ½ cup milk or soy milk (zinc, calcium, magnesium, B complex)
or
Whole grain bread with a nut or seed butter (calcium, thiamin, zinc, B complex)
with
A boiled egg (or 4 ounces of broiled or pan-broiled fish) (protein, essential fatty acids)
or
Low-fat organic yogurt (calcium/lactobacillus—good bacteria). Do not eat yogurt if you have a persistent yeast problem.
One cup only of organic coffee (caffeine boost) or ginger tea

*Mid-morning snack*

Organic beef or chicken bullion (protein, zinc)
or
Raw carrots (vitamin A) and celery

## LUNCH

Organic garden salad made with dark leafy greens, yellow vegetables, red peppers, mushrooms, and any other raw vegetables (high levels of many vitamins and minerals).
Broiled salmon or tuna fish (zinc, calcium, thiamin, protein, "good" fats)
One cup whole cooked grain, such as brown rice or buckwheat (B complex) or baked potato (vitamin C)
yogurt, 1 cup (calcium)
fresh peas (niacin) or steamed greens (calcium, vitamin C, B vitamins) and carrots (vitamin A)

## DINNER

Large organic garden salad (vitamins, minerals)
Four ounces lean meat, fish, or poultry (zinc, calcium, thiamin, protein, "good" fats)
One cup of a cooked whole grain (B complex) or a potato or yam (vitamins C and A)

Steamed veggies (several vitamins and minerals)
One piece of fresh fruit (vitamins)

***Evening snack***

Low fat yogurt (calcium)
A small handful of dry roasted nuts and seeds (many minerals, especially zinc and protein)
Figs (potassium, calcium, magnesium, iron)
For a healthy, sex-boosting snack, mix organic dry roasted seeds and/or nuts in yogurt or kefir (yogurt drink), along with a few pieces of dried figs.

## Libido Killers

Eat natural. That's easy enough. You are probably already eating a lot of the "right stuff" without even thinking about it. But there's more. If you want to achieve truly vibrant sexual health, you should consider some don'ts as well. Again, sexual function and overall nutrition health are linked. You don't have to go macrobiotic, but here is a list of foods that are known to drag you down.

***Simple Sugars and Refined Starches***

Simple sugars and starches are deadly to the libido. That "rush" of energy after eating a candy bar or glazed doughnut is deceptive. It lasts all of fifteen minutes to half an hour and is the exact opposite of a true turn-on tonic. The rush comes from a sharp rise in your blood sugar levels, but the high soon switches direction and heads downward. You are left exhausted. Over time this pattern leads to a condition in which blood sugar levels are chronically low (hypoglycemia). You always feel depleted, emotionally unstable, and constantly tired—too tired for sex.

***Saturated Fat***

A lot of confusion surrounds the subject of dietary fats. The problems arise when we eat the *wrong type of fat.* Certain fats are needed for optimum sexual functioning. These fats help store the fat-soluble vitamins A, D, and E, all of which are key to smooth sexual function. Fat is also the most concentrated source of body energy and is an essential source of energy on the cellular level.

The right fats are called "essential fatty acids," which must come from the foods you eat, specifically *unhydrogenated* vegetable oils, such as flax seed (the best), safflower, canola, wheat germ, sesame seed, walnut, olive, and soybean. Other foods rich in essential fatty acids include peanuts, olives, nuts, chicken, and fish. Omega-3 fatty acids, found in tuna and salmon, can lower LDL cholesterol and triglyceride levels, thereby helping you maintain healthy heart function—another essential for a healthy sex life.

Bad fats are "hydrogenated," which means that they solidify at room temperature. Since your body cannot absorb these fats, they deposit as plaque along your blood vessel walls, eventually causing artery and heart disease and poor sexual function. Hydrogenated fats include all animal fats (those found in dairy products and meats), lard, shellfish, cooked coconut oil, and palm oil. However, frying even "good" fats will turn them "bad." The high level of heat involved in the frying process alters their chemical structure so that they transform into hydrogenated or saturated fats. Another problem food is margarine. Though we hear advertisements recommending it as a healthy substitute for butter, it is loaded with harmful trans-fatty acids, which, like saturated oils and fats, cannot be used by the body. All these are the prime culprits behind the high cholesterol levels that lead to restricted blood flow. If your sex organs and glands cannot receive sufficient blood, they are not able to function or produce enough hormones.

## NUTRITION TIPS FOR BETTER SEX

The following easy-to-follow nutritional tips give you some guidelines for eating right and enjoying the energy and health you need to enjoy great sex:

- Include fresh fruits and vegetables, whole grains, lean meats, fish, and plenty of pure water.
- Avoid refined, processed, canned, frozen, and precooked foods.
- Watch how much shellfish you eat. They contain essential vitamins and minerals, but they are high in cholesterol.
- Whenever possible, choose unprocessed and organic whole

foods. Eat free-range animal products—that is, meat and dairy products from animals raised on pesticide- and hormone-free diets and in natural surroundings.

- If you are lactose-intolerant, try goat milk products or yogurt and kefir. If you prefer a dairy-free diet or are allergic to dairy altogether, substitute soy milk and other soybean products.
- Avoid drinking tap water. It is full of chemicals, and, on occasion, harmful microbes. Bottled water is good, or try using filters. Some of them fit right onto your faucet.
- Watch your intake of alcohol. One or two glasses of red wine a day, though, have been shown in recent studies to lower cholesterol.
- Avoid carbonated sodas. They are full of either sugar or artificial sweeteners and, sometimes, caffeine.
- Watch that caffeine! Black tea, chocolate, colas, coffee, and some over-the-counter medications (including menstrual pain

## ❧ ORGANIC YOGURT

Yogurt that contains live lactobacillus acidophilis cultures can help prevent recurrent common vaginal infections by promoting the presence of "good" bacteria. The recommended daily dose is about five ounces. However, if you suffer from a severe overgrowth of the yeast known as candida albicans, it will actually thrive on yogurt cultures. If this is your problem, consult your health-care provider. Other dietary measures that discourage candida infections include avoiding sugar, chocolate, refined starches, and alcohol.

---

Most menstrual cramps are caused by too much estrogen and too little progesterone, and caffeine aggravates the problem by interfering with the proper metabolism of estrogen. Caffeine also has a negative effect on the pancreas, causing fluctuations in blood sugar levels that can create or aggravate the symptoms of premenstrual syndrome (PMS), breast sensitivity, and menstrual cramps.

relief formulas) all contain caffeine. Even decaffeinated coffee—unless it is decaffeinated by a water process—contains methylxanthines, a family of chemicals that includes caffeine.

To wean yourself off coffee and other caffeinated beverages without experiencing uncomfortable withdrawal symptoms, decrease your daily intake gradually. If you want to drink decaffeinated coffee, look for a label that says "water process."

Another option is to limit yourself to one cup of organic coffee a day. Or you can drink a good substitute, ginger tea, which has similar stimulating and energizing effects. To make ginger tea, grate a few teaspoons of raw ginger root into a quart of water. Bring almost to a boil—boiling will destroy its potency—then simmer for ten minutes.

- Eliminate white sugar and products made with white sugar. Try honey, fruit juice or concentrate, or maple syrup. If you are prone to yeast infections or low blood sugar, eliminate sweeteners altogether.
- Stay away from saturated fats and cholesterol-rich foods. That includes fatty meats, whole milk products (especially cheese), most baked goods, all fast foods (doughnuts, hot dogs, potato chips, french fries, etc.).
- Do not fry foods. Get all the nutritional benefits from your vegetables by steaming them lightly. Broil, pan broil, roast, or bake meats.
- Use sea salt sparingly. Use small amounts of salt in the preparation of your food and sprinkle it lightly to taste on your meals. Adequate levels of salt do ensure our optimum strength and sexual energy, but you want to keep your sodium levels from getting too high. Use natural herbs, spices, and lemon juice to add further flavor. Avoid commercially packaged seasoning preparations. Also avoid processed foods, which can contain large quantities of sodium.
- Eat zinc-rich sunflower, pumpkin, and sesame seeds to support your sex-gland function. Many ancient cultures have prized these seeds because they support sex hormone production, especially for males. Gypsies have been eating pumpkin seeds for centuries in order to boost hormone levels and maintain healthy prostate function. Women in ancient Babylonia nibbled all day long on sesame seed and honey confections to increase their libi-

dos and fertility. Modern-day French women snack on the same concoction to boost their sexual vitality. You can do the same by filling a small plastic bag with seeds and carrying them wherever you go, so you always have a healthy, sex-boosting snack on hand.

Finally, try to eat smaller amounts of food more frequently. In fact, eating less overall is one of the best strategies for sexual longevity.

Be kind to yourself when it comes to your diet. Don't make changes all at once. Instead, take your time, gradually introducing new foods and eliminating old, non-nutritious favorites, only as you feel ready. You will soon discover, much to your surprise, that your taste in food actually transforms, as your palate refines and becomes more sensitive. Natural, nutritious foods will begin to taste more delicious, and those loaded with sugar, simple starches, unhealthy fats, and chemical additives will lose their appeal.

As you grow more in touch with your body's needs, you will come to view appetites for certain foods as signals from your body telling you what nutritional elements you need in order to enjoy optimum health, sexual health included.

In fact, all the information that follows this chapter is designed to further this goal of joining mind and body in perfect synchrony, so that you can create for yourself the most satisfying and passionate sex life possible.

## QUIT SMOKING

Quitting smoking will work wonders for your sex life, because smoking reduces testosterone levels, thereby lowering the sex drive in both sexes. Smoking also decreases the action of nerve chemicals that control erections, and it constricts blood flow to the sex organs of men and women. That means, if you smoke, your libido suffers, as does the intensity of your orgasms.

# 2

# THE HERB CONNECTION

Herbology, the study of the healing and strengthening effects of medicinal plants, is the oldest form of medicine known to man. In contrast to modern medicine, which is barely a century old, the use of nature as a pharmacy can be traced back to the civilizations of Rome, Greece, Assyria, Babylonia, even to Sumerian times. Over many centuries, painstaking experiments with flowers, weeds, plants, roots, leaves, and seeds have yielded a stock of natural medicines that prevent and heal many ailments.

From the very beginning, a primary focus of herbology was discovering natural remedies that promote a healthier and more intensely pleasurable sex life. Since recorded time, women seeking to fulfill their erotic potential and increase their fertility and men desiring greater sexual potency have relied on the powerful benefits of herbal treatments.

The advent of modern drugs—vaccines, antibiotics, and other pharmaceuticals—cast the science of healing herbs into the shadows. All that is currently changing, though. In recent years the pendulum has swung back toward natural remedies. More and more people have grown dissatisfied with modern medicine because of the unpleasant, potentially harmful side effects. Many are seeking out less expensive preventive methods that work with the body's own resources to strengthen resistance to disease and improve overall health.

Time-tested natural herbal teas and fluid extracts are being rediscovered, including botanical supplements in tablets and capsules. New ways of toning and healing our bodies through plant remedies are also being explored. People are finally realizing that no single body function can be isolated from the others, just as good general health and good sexual health are inextricably linked. Therefore, all natural herbal remedies that improve your overall health will naturally benefit your sex life. And the reverse is equally true.

Benjamin Franklin once said, "An ounce of prevention is worth a pound of cure." That adage holds just as true today. Herbal medicine, coupled with sound nutrition, still delivers the most powerful protection there is. Plant remedies—prepared as teas, decoctions, tinctures (fluid extracts), tablets, or capsules—promote overall wellness by maintaining the body's harmonious balance, strength, and optimum energy levels. The toning herbs described in this chapter support, stimulate, and enhance the function of the sex organs and glands so that you can enjoy a lifetime's worth of youthful vigor and passion.

Still, less than one percent of the 250,000-odd plant species on earth have been studied for medicinal properties. Studies to verify the healing powers of herbs cost many millions of dollars. What drug company would underwrite costs to verify the strengthening and healing properties of a substance that grows wild—a substance they cannot patent and sell for profit?

This is why many of the claims made for herbal healing are based on anecdotal clinical evidence rather than on scientifically sanctioned double-blind studies. Although more scientifically approved studies of herbs are being conducted today than ever before, users of herbs often have to rely on the testimony of numerous modern-day natural practitioners, as well as on records handed down from ancient healers, reporting the beneficial effects of various herbs on their many thousands of patients.

For our purposes, all the evidence that has been gathered supports the contention made by millions: Nature's herbal cupboard overflows with valuable plant remedies that can help you counter the sexual doldrums, increase your potency, and enjoy more intense, longer-lasting orgasms. The primrose path to the sex life you've always dreamed of is strewn with flower petals, after all, as well as with roots, leaves, barks, and weeds.

Until relatively recently if you wanted to use herbs, you had to brew the remedies yourself. Though some enjoy experimenting with their own remedies, you no longer have to make them from scratch. A wide variety of herbal remedies are now available, in single and compound formulas.

Whether you purchase your remedies at the store or through mail order or decide to try your hand as an herbalist, use the following instructions to guide you.

## TYPES OF HERBAL REMEDY PREPARATIONS

### *Basic Infusion Recipe*

An infusion is a tea made from an herb, usually the leaves, flowers, and some berries. If you are making an herbal tea, use pure spring water, distilled water, or filtered water. Bring the water to a boil, then pour the water *over* the herb, and allow it to steep in a covered container for five to ten minutes. The standard formula for an infusion is one teaspoon of dried herb to one cup of boiling water, although you might use less herb material if the herb is very strong, more if it is weak. If you are using green (fresh) herbs, use one-half ounce of herb to one pint of boiling water. Remember not to boil the herb *with* the water, since boiling can rob herbal flowers and leaves of their medicinal properties.

Strain out the herbs and drink while warm. (If you prefer a sweeter-tasting tea, add one-half teaspoon of either cardamom powder or licorice root powder to the herb and steep together. You won't need to do this if fennel or licorice are part of your tonic.) The usual dose for a tea is three to four cups a day.

### *Decoction*

A decoction is a tea made with barks, roots, branches, and berries. It's stronger than an infusion, and the herbal materials are boiled in water for ten to thirty minutes to extract their medicinal properties. The longer you boil, the more medicinal properties you extract. However, the boiling time entirely depends on which herbal ingredients you are using. Strain out the boiled plant parts before drinking. The usual dose for a decoction is three to four cups a day.

### *Fluid Tinctures*

Chop the herb finely and add one ounce of herb to one pint of lab-proof alcohol, which is available in some pharmacies (*do not* use rubbing alcohol), or vodka. Lab-proof alcohol is preferable. Shake daily. After two weeks, strain and use according to instructions. The usual dose is one teaspoonful or ten to fifteen drops diluted in half a cup of warm water, three to four times a day. If you buy commercially prepared tinctures (also known as fluid extracts), follow the dose instructions on the bottle label.

### *Capsules*

Almost any herb can be powdered and placed in a gelatin capsule. Of course, it's far more convenient to purchase the capsules, but you can powder herbs yourself and place them in capsules. The standard capsule size is referred to as "00." Capsules allow you mobility. You can swallow them with water wherever you are, but you still have the option of opening the capsules, pouring out the contents, and adding hot water for tea. The usual dosage for capsules is three to four capsules a day, taken in divided doses. That can vary, depending on the herb, so follow the dose instructions on the bottle label.

### *Guidelines for Making Your Own Remedies*

1. Herbs packaged in tea bags tend to have lost much of their beneficial properties by the time you buy them. If you are able to gather the fresh herb yourself, try to use it immediately.
2. You can buy dried herbs or dry them yourself in tightly sealed glass or ceramic containers. Either way, the container will help to preserve their freshness.
3. Use pure water and organic ingredients in making your remedies.
4. Do not use aluminum wares for making any herbal preparations. Preparations made in aluminum utensils, which leach aluminum into the preparation, can cause stomach ulcers. Enamel, glass, and stainless steel pots are best.

## Principles of Herbal Healing

Though herbs are safer than pharmaceutical drugs, in order to receive their full strengthening and healing benefits, follow these basic healing principles.

- Different herbs are best used during specific times of the year. Roots and barks are considered most appropriate to use in wintertime, while leaves and flowers are best used during summertime.
- Dry herbs should not be used after one year, since they lose 50 percent of their effectiveness, even if you picked and dried them yourself. Roots, barks, and some berries can be kept and used longer than most leaves.
- Most herbs should be taken on an empty stomach. The usual recommendation is at least a half hour before eating or two hours after a meal. Follow this procedure unless specifically instructed otherwise.
- Unless specifically indicated, women should not take herbs during their menstrual periods or when pregnant.

## Tonic Herbs

Herbs are usually divided into several basic groups. *Tonic* herbs revive energy and stimulate function. *Nutritive* herbs soothe, calm, and build. *Carminative* herbs expel gas, stimulate stomach secretions, and help the stomach to absorb and assimilate nutrients. *Astringent* and *disinfectant* herbs cleanse, eliminate, and break down excess matter, such as the excess mucus created by an ulcerated area.

For our purposes, which are to prevent health problems that could short-circuit your sex life and to make your dream of sexual rejuvenation a reality, your best bet is to use tonic herbs that strengthen and stimulate the function of your sex organs and glands.

Tonic herbs are generally nontoxic—the safest of all herbs—and usually can be taken over the long term. They can be ingested either individually or in compound remedies that include several herbs working together to strengthen and tone your body. Tonics can be consumed in many forms—capsule, tincture, decoction, or as an infusion or tea. The following list describes the most commonly used tonic herbs for increasing sexual health and creating supercharged lovers.

### *Black Cohosh* (Cimicifuga racemosa)

Also known as squaw root, this popular traditional Native American herb was used by tribal women to speed up childbirth. Black cohosh boosts estrogen production and ovulation by enabling the transport of estrogen throughout the body, and it also acts to strengthen the uterus. It is used by young women as one of the most effective remedies for bringing on delayed menstrual flow and for relieving symptoms of difficult menstrual periods, as well as by older women to relieve the symptoms of menopause.

*DOSE:* For a tea, boil two teaspoons of dried roots in one pint of water. Take two or three teaspoons six times a day; take five to thirty drops of the fluid extract in one cup water once a day; or take two to three capsules a day. If sexual desire is low or you are menopausal, take four capsules a day.

*SAFETY ISSUES:* Do not use if you are pregnant. Very large doses can cause symptoms of poisoning. Women whose blood sugar levels are low could experience an aggravation of symptoms.

### *Borage* (Borago officinalis)

The leaves of this plant, with exquisite blue starlike flowers, taste like cucumber and have been used since the days of the ancient Greeks for a wide variety of ailments, particularly for depression and nervous tension. This herb is a rich source of calcium and potassium, minerals important to the nervous system and for calming and strengthening the heart. Borage also tones and stimulates the adrenal glands, which traditional Eastern medicine views as the prime source of sexual vitality.

Borage oil, taken in capsules, pills, or as part of a compound supplement, is an effective treatment for the symptoms of menopause.

DOSE: Follow dose instructions on the bottle label for borage oil. You can also make a tea, using either one teaspoon of dried flowers or two to three teaspoons of dried leaves steeped in a half cup of hot water.

SAFETY ISSUES: Do not use for over a month at a time.

### *Chamomile* (Anthemis nobilis)

Known for its soothing, sedative, and harmless tranquilizing effects, chamomile tea stimulates menstrual flow (when taken cold) and helps relieve PMS and menstrual cramps. Chamomile contains calcium in an easily absorbed form, plus a volatile oil and glucoside with relaxing qualities. All of this makes chamomile a wonderful herb for menstruating, perimenopausal, and menopausal women, and anyone of any age who can benefit from a natural tranquilizer that soothes the nerves and the digestive tract.

Chamomile also boasts natural antibiotic properties. Chamomile steam baths are said to ease difficulty in men's urination due to enlarged prostate. Chamomile comes loose and dried, in tea bags, capsules, and tinctures, and is widely available.

DOSE: Drink the tea freely, using one teaspoon of dried leaves per cup of water, and follow the dose instructions on capsule and tincture bottles.

SAFETY ISSUES: None, unless you're using a homeopathic substance. Wait two to three hours after taking the homeopathic remedy before using chamomile in any form.

### *Corn Silk* (Zea mays *or* Stigmata maidis)

The yellowish, fine "threads" that cover the ears of corn were a popular remedy for bladder complaints in the old days and later were prescribed by doctors as a diuretic and to relieve cystitis and even gonorrhea in both sexes. Corn silk is still prescribed today and is available in loose or dried form, in capsules and tinctures.

DOSE: Follow dose instructions on the bottle label. You can also drink the tea freely to relieve bouts of cystitis.

SAFETY ISSUES: None.

## *Cramp Bark* (Viburnum opulus)

Native Americans made pills and medicinal plasters from cramp bark, and they smoked the bark as a substitute for tobacco. Cramp bark is a powerful antispasmodic, making it a great way of regulating and relaxing the ovaries and uterus, thereby easing uterine pains and cramps. Some natural health-care providers recommend it in tea form to prevent miscarriage.

*DOSE:* The usual dose is two to three cups of the hot tea per day to relieve cramps. A half cup of strong tea will relieve cramps in twenty minutes. If you use the fluid extract, take ten to twenty drops three times a day.

*SAFETY ISSUES:* None.

## *Damiana* (Turnera diffusa)

This shrub grows wild in Southern California, Mexico, and Texas. The peoples indigenous to the above areas have used damiana leaves since antiquity to relieve nervous and muscular weakness, both of which can weaken orgasms. They even use it to firm women's breasts and normalize their size, either reducing or enlarging them. In turn-of-the-century America, the fluid extract of damiana or pills made from the leaves were used as a remedy for impotence. Damiana is still prescribed today to relieve all of the above conditions. Scientists generally agree that damiana has a tonic effect on the reproductive organs in both sexes through its action on the spinal cord. It corrects both nervous exhaustion and sexual weakness, especially when both conditions are caused by sexual excess. Though damiana's chemical composition is not entirely known, its oils are thought to stimulate the reproductive and nervous systems, as well as enhance circulation, thereby priming your body for more intense sexual pleasure.

*DOSE:* Damiana is available in capsules and tinctures. If you use the tea, pour half a pint of boiling water over one teaspoon of either the dried berry and leaf or the powder. Steep until cool then take one teaspoon three times a day. Individual needs for damiana vary widely. You can take between two to six capsules (each contains 480 mg per capsule) a day.

*SAFETY ISSUES:* None.

### *Dong Quai* (Angelica)

An excellent tonic for female sex glands and organs, this Chinese herb is also called "the female ginseng," because it is one of the most effective herbs for enhancing female sexual function and general health, nourishing and supporting the ovaries and hormone production throughout a woman's life, as well as supplying her abundantly with iron. It also contains high levels of vitamin E, balances and maintains hormone levels, enhances the blood vessels and arteries, and boosts the immune system. Dong quai is particularly helpful for increasing the libidos of perimenopausal and menopausal women. For this reason, dong quai has long been used by Asian healers to cure many female disorders but most commonly for relieving menopausal symptoms and painful menstrual cramping.

Dong quai is widely available in health food stores, Chinese herbal pharmacies, and through mail order in capsule and tincture forms. It is frequently found in compound tonics prescribed by both Chinese and Western herbalists. Some compound formulas combine dong quai with chaste berry, another libido enhancer that works in a similar manner to balance hormone levels, thereby ensuring healthy functioning of the sex organs and glands, and easing premenstrual syndrome (PMS), menopausal symptoms, and other endocrine gland–related disorders.

*DOSE:* Unless you are trying to correct a specific problem or are experiencing strong menopausal symptoms, you don't need to take dong quai more than one to two times per month—and never during the menstrual cycle. Standard dose is one teaspoon of the fluid extract three times a day. In its other forms, follow the dose instructions on the bottle label.

*SAFETY ISSUES:* Though it is generally considered safe, some of dong quai's chemical components can interact with sunlight and cause a rash or severe sunburn.

### *Echinacea* (Echinacea angustifolia)

This extract from the purple coneflower, a daisylike plant common to the American plains, is a known immune-system toner and lymph-system stimulant. Echinacea has come into the spotlight in the past several years because of the increasing number of people complaining of chronic fatigue and a variety of immunodeficient diseases.

Echinacea works by stimulating stem cells in bone marrow and lymphatic tissue. Less known is this powerful herb's ability to relieve urinary frequency due to an inflammed prostate gland (prostatitis).

*DOSE:* Echinacea comes in a wide variety of forms. Some homeopathic doctors even prescribe injections of homeopathic echinacea formulations. Usually it is taken in fluid extract form, less often in capsule form. The usual dose for the extract is a quarter to half teaspoon three to four times a day. Otherwise, follow the dose instructions on the bottle label.

*SAFETY ISSUES:* None. The latest studies state that echinacea is safe when taken on a long-term basis, but if you are healthy and your immune system is operating well, you do not need it. If your immune system is impaired, you can feel confident in taking this herb for as long as needed.

## *Evening Primrose Oil* (Oenothera biennis)

Except for mother's milk, evening primrose is the richest known source of both linoleic acid and gamma-linoleic acid (GLA). Both are crucial to optimum sexual function and heightened sex-hormore response, including estrogen and testosterone, because hormones are made by the body from these essential fatty acids. The oil extracted from the evening primrose seeds also helps the body manufacture prostaglandins (PGs), which regulate a wide range of body functions including blood pressure and cholesterol levels.

Evening primrose oil is mainly recommended for women to maintain peak hormonal levels. If you don't have enough PGs, you can suffer from such sex-function-related problems as PMS and menstrual cramps. Men who lack sufficient PGs may produce low amounts of ejaculate.

This oil is also effective as an anti-inflammatory. Initial experiments proved its action only when evening primrose oil was administered by injection. But recent research suggests that when it's taken in enteric-coated tablets (which enables it to bypass the intestinal tract and deliver its ingredients directly to the bloodstream), evening primrose helps relieve PMS and other inflammatory conditions affecting the female organs and glands.

Some researchers also consider evening primrose oil to be a good preventative and a cure for cysts in the breasts and ovaries.

*DOSE:* When combined with vitamin $B_6$ and vitamin E, evening primrose oil becomes a powerful weapon against premenstrual tension (PMS). Take six 500 mg capsules of evening primrose oil daily in three doses of 1,000 mg each, about a week before menstruation. At the same time, take 50 mg of $B_6$ once a day, along with 200 to 600 mg of vitamin E a day, split into two or three doses.

If this program is followed for a few months, it also helps correct overlong, overly profuse menstrual periods.

If you are using the tincture, take twenty to forty drops in water as needed.

*SAFETY ISSUES:* High doses (2,500 mg three times a day) for too long a period (more than six to eight months) can lead to fibroid tumors.

### *Fenugreek* (Trigonella foenumgraecum)

These tasty, nutritious seeds are found in various East Indian, Pakastani, and African dishes, but fenugreek was first prized by the ancient peoples of Asia and those who lived on the shores of the Mediterranean as a valuable antipollutant for the body. Pollutants are often stored in the mucus and fatty tissue that surround sex organs and glands, thereby impeding circulation and healthy function. These toxins and mucus can also create cholesterol plaque on the blood vessels, impairing circulation and thus lowering libido and making it difficult to get and sustain an erection. Needless to say, fenugreek's antipollutant action is even more essential in today's postindustrial world.

Fenugreek is also rich in an oil that contains high levels of vitamins A and D, as well as trimethylamine, which acts as a sex hormone in frogs. Turkish women snack on a mixture of powdered fenugreek seeds and honey to rejuvenate their sexuality and sweeten their breath. Turkish men eat this mixture to enhance their potency.

DOSE: Fenugreek seed can be brewed into a tea that is a wonderful natural medicine for an impressive array of ailments, including helping the body discharge the excess mucus and the toxins trapped in it. Steep two teaspoons of the seeds in a cup of boiling water for five minutes. Strain and add honey and/or lemon or lime juice. Drink freely.

SAFETY ISSUES: None.

## *Feverfew* (Tanacetum parthenium)

Nature's headache and fever remedy is fast becoming one of the most sought-after alternative medicines for pain relief because its anti-inflammatory effect is similar to that of aspirin—without the side effects. Studies have confirmed that among feverfew's benefits are relief from menstrual cramps.

DOSE: Feverfew is available in loose or dried form, tea bags, capsules, and tinctures. However, for any preparation to be effective, it must contain about .25 to .5 mg of parthenolide, feverfew's active ingredient. A recent analysis of thirty-five different commercial preparations found that they contained widely varying amounts of parthenolide, with some even showing no traces of it. So, the best form of feverfew is standardized capsules that deliver a consistent amount of its active principles. Take two tablets or capsules a day.

SAFETY ISSUES: If you use feverfew consistently for more than four to six weeks, you risk developing cold sores, fever blisters, or a skin rash.

## *Garlic* (Allium sativum)

Whole garlic contains an antibiotic oil and is also rich in vitamins essential for optimum sexual health: vitamin A, thiamine, riboflavin, and niacin. A close relative of the onion, garlic has a history of service to mankind as ancient and honorable as that of any plant. The intense smell of garlic may ward off potential lovers (along with vampires), but among its many wonderful benefits are its ability to lower blood pressure, thin blood, aid circulation, detoxify, and lower cholesterol and triglycerides in the blood, thereby making it essential for healthy sexual functioning. Researchers at Tulane University discovered that total cholesterol and low-density (bad) cholesterol are reduced after a twelve-week regime of 1½ cloves of garlic or a 900 mg capsule of powdered garlic daily.

Garlic also boosts immune function, helps relieve PMS and bring on menstrual flow, and has an antifungal action.

*DOSE:* Commercial garlic preparations should contain a daily dose of at least 10 mg of allin, garlic's active medicinal ingredient. You can also eat this pungent bulb freely, with the ideal amount being about one clove a day. Use it as a seasoning for your food.

Most brands of garlic capsules, tablets, and liquids are specially processed to be odorless. Recommended dose for optimum effectiveness ranges from 800 to 1,600 mg per day.

*SAFETY ISSUES:* Too much garlic can irritate the intestinal tract, and studies using rats found that very large amounts of garlic over very long periods of time caused anemia, weight loss, and failure to grow.

### *Ginger* (Zingiber officinale)

Ginger is native to southern Asia and has been used in China for thousands of years for medicinal purposes. Today, virtually all tropical countries cultivate this root—particularly Jamaica—for its use as a delicious spice and its wonderful healing properties.

Ginger poultices are used by traditional Asian healers to relieve congestion anywhere in the body. Like aspirin, but without the side effects, ginger also helps prevent strokes and heart failure. Jamaicans use their famous homegrown ginger to heal many ailments as well as to increase sexual potency.

Ginger root is classified as a stimulant that jump-starts the endocrine glands, key to maintaining optimum sexual desire and function. It is also an effective anti-inflammatory and combats motion sickness. Recent studies confirm that ginger lowers cholesterol levels even more effectively than onion or garlic.

Most people use ginger root to relieve nausea and indigestion. But this invigorating root increases circulation and heat anywhere in the body, making it an effective menstruation promoter, migraine headache and cold and flu reliever, and a delicious and energizing replacement for coffee.

DOSE: Ginger root can be grated and used as a condiment or brewed as a tea, which can be drunk freely. The fresh root is probably the most effective, but if the whole root is not available at your local health food store or Asian grocery, you can find ginger in capsules and tinctures. Follow dose instructions on the bottle label. Studies generally use one gram of powdered dry ginger root, but in India people commonly eat eight to ten grams a day. You can experiment to see how much relieves your nausea, indigestion, or circulation problems.

SAFETY ISSUES: If large amounts are taken on an empty stomach, ginger can irritate the gastrointestinal tract. Studies have found that taking as much as six grams of dried powdered root at a time, over prolonged periods, can damage the intestinal lining and possibly lead to ulcers.

## *Gingko Biloba*

Also known as the maidenhair tree, *Gingko biloba* barely survived the Ice Age to become one of the oldest plant species on earth. A longtime staple of Chinese medicine, it is generally prescribed to stimulate the brain and boost short-term memory. *Gingko biloba* is also an effective anti-oxidant and free-radical scavenger. In fluid extract form, gingko has become one of today's most prescribed medicines in Europe and America for poor circulation and for improving mental function. It does this by dilating and toning the blood vessels, thereby improving blood flow, which helps the brain use oxygen and glucose more efficiently and increases the rate of nerve transmissions. Gingko also improves microcirculation and peripheral circulation of blood to the extremities. Since the penis is an extremity that contains many tiny blood vessels, if you increase its blood and energy circulation, potency naturally increases, which means that gingko produces better erections in men and helps women's sex organs engorge more fully with blood.

A recent study conducted at the University of California at San Francisco indicates that gingko can correct the lack of sexual desire commonly experienced by people taking antidepressants such as Prozac, Zoloft, and Paxil. Two 60 mg capsules were taken by thirty-seven men and women, all of whom had experienced loss of libido and delayed orgasm from antidepressants. After taking gingko, 86 percent reported significant improvement in their sex lives. Studies have also confirmed gingko's effectiveness in relieving the congestion of premenstrual tension.

In a recent German study, twenty men with severe impotence took an 80 mg capsule three times a day for nine months. Every participant reported spontaneous erections and marked increase in hardness.

*DOSE:* *Gingko biloba* comes as a standardized fluid extract at 24 percent potency, and in capsule form. Unless otherwise directed by your health-care provider, the standard dose is ten drops after each meal, or one 60 mg capsule in the morning and one in the evening.

*SAFETY ISSUES:* If you are allergic to gingko, you could experience a mild skin rash. Other possible side effects, which are not really harmful, include increased warmth in the extremities, a slight flush on the skin, or a tender headache. These result from increased oxygen and blood flow and are not at all harmful.

Do not take *Gingko biloba* if you have been diagnosed with a blood-clotting disorder or if you are pregnant or nursing. Gingko leaf extract is quite safe. However, ingesting or touching the fruit pulp can cause such side effects as vomiting, diarrhea, headaches, and itchy skin irritations.

## *Ginseng Root, Panax* (Panax quinquefolia *or* Panax schinseng)

This venerable herb is a true toner and energizer that restores overall strength, muscle tone, and vitality in those who are chronically fatigued or have been weakened by illness. Ginseng proponents make numerous claims for its healing and strengthening abilities, including its ability to maintain optimum and steady blood pressure, blood sugar, metabolism, and energy levels. All these body systems are involved in sexual desire and performance, which is one reason why ginseng has enjoyed a centuries-old reputation in Asia and the Americas as an herb that supports sexual function. Ginseng also directly benefits the sex organs and glands. Although ginseng is usually thought of as a man's herb, it also strengthens women's sex organs and glands, thereby enhancing female sexual desire, especially women with low testosterone levels. And contrary to popular myth, women can take either panax or Siberian ginseng.

The panax forms of ginseng are more active than the Siberian form and are better suited to increasing sexual desire. Siberian ginseng is used more for increasing mental clarity than sex drive.

Panax ginseng is traditionally prescribed as a rejuvenating tonic, energizer, and miracle worker for the sex organs and glands because of its known strengthening effect on the endocrine system. In animal studies, panax ginseng has increased testosterone levels while decreasing prostate weight, suggesting that it can protect men from impotency and inflammation and swelling of the prostate gland. Ginseng also has been shown to support growth of the testicles in young men, increase sperm formation, and accelerate ovary growth in young women. It also helps to preserve the health of female reproductive tissues following a hysterectomy or menopause.

Panax ginseng is naturally found in both Asia and North America. The beauty of panax ginseng is that it aids toleration of stress, which is why it's classified as an adaptogen. Adaptogen herbs can be taken for as long as you like.

*DOSE:* Ginseng is best taken in the morning because of its stimulating action. Various roots differ widely in their effectiveness. Generally, the more expensive the root, the more effectively it works with less risk of irritation. You can either chew the root, drink the tea, take the powder or mix it in your food, or swallow capsules.

The dose depends on the content of ginsenoside, the active ingredient in panax ginseng. Choose your brand carefully, selecting one that is standardized to give you at least .5 percent of ginsenosides. Solar Ray is one of the best formulations of ginseng available. Take one capsule a day to maintain ginsenoside levels in your blood stream. One dose of the standardized extract—ten to fifteen drops—will do the same.

*SAFETY ISSUES:* Ginseng has the advantage of being perfectly safe over long-term use. But if you suffer from high blood pressure, it could rise when you take this root. Women taking panax ginseng may experience breast tenderness. Reduce the dose and the pain will cease.

### *Ginseng, Siberian* (Eleutherococcus senticosus)

A close cousin of panax ginseng, Siberian ginseng is also a good energizer and stress reliever (whether that stress has physical or emotional causes). Siberian ginseng also tones the adrenals, thereby strengthening the sex organs and glands in both sexes, and is well suited for long-term use. However, it is less effective as a sex tonic than as a way to improve mental clarity.

*DOSE:* You can drink ginseng tea, chew the root, take capsules or tablets, ingest the extract, or mix it into various beverages. A recent study found that the extract and powder forms are more effective than fresh sliced ginseng, its juice, or tea, particularly if that extract is made from high-grade roots. Take one capsule or ten to fifteen drops of the fluid extract per day.

*SAFETY ISSUES:* None.

### *Licorice Root* (Glycyrrhiza glabra)

Known as "the great harmonizer" in Chinese medicine, this tasty root sweetens many tonic formulas and is also a great anti-inflammatory, toner, and energizer for the entire body, particularly for the adrenal glands, mainly by virtue of its most active medicinal ingredient, glycyrrhizin. Licorice root also normalizes estrogen metabolism, inhibiting estrogen action when the levels are too high and boosting its action when levels are too low. It also has anti-allergic properties.

Many health-minded ex-smokers chew on this root to calm their tobacco cravings, at the same time that they tone their organs and promote better gum health. Some traditional cultures use licorice root to increase fertility.

*DOSE:* Licorice root is available in whole form in health food stores and Asian herbal stores. It is also widely available in tea, capsule, and tincture form. The dosage is based on the content level of its active ingredients, particularly glycyrrhizin, and also on your blood pressure. Licorice can increase blood pressure, so you need to monitor what works for you and what doesn't. The standard dose is one to two capsules a day.

*SAFETY ISSUES:* Licorice root can increase blood pressure; do not take if you have hypertension, a history of renal failure, or use digitalis preparations. If more than three grams are taken per day for more than six weeks, it can cause water and sodium retention, hypertension, and other problems. You can counter these possible side effects by sticking to a high-potassium, low-sodium diet.

### *Onion* (Allium cepa)

The onion is one of the oldest vegetables known to man.. In ancient times people placed slices of onion around the home, believing that its pungent aroma would ward off evil spirits and diseases. In fact, some people follow this custom today, destroying the peeled, bruised, or cut bulb (and whatever diseases and evil spirits it has trapped) after a few hours. Researchers have found scientific evidence to support that practice: onions produce an electrical field similar to that produced by penicillin.

For herbalists, the onion is similar to garlic in its health benefits, although its action is generally not as powerful. Onion juice is an effective diuretic and a valuable aid to your sex life because it normalizes blood pressure, especially if it's too high, and helps restore sexual potency.

*DOSE:* Doses for medicinal purposes usually range from a quarter to a cup of chopped onion a day. You can eat onion freely, but be sure to freshen your breath (try parsley) afterward.

*SAFETY ISSUES:* None.

### *Red Raspberry* (Rubus idaeus)

Raspberry leaves are particularly helpful for women because raspberry strengthens and tones the uterus. It relieves almost all kinds of female problems because it also has a wonderful soothing action, and it is one of the few herbs that can be used throughout pregnancy.

Among raspberry's many benefits to women are reducing overly heavy menstrual flow, easing uterine cramps and labor pains, and helping to counter prolapsed uterus. The tea is said to help prevent miscarriage and morning sickness. Red raspberry also has astringent and cleansing properties, making it an excellent herb for postpartum recovery and for enriching breast milk. The tea also makes an excellent douche for common vaginitis and fungal infections.

DOSE: Red raspberry is available in bulk, tea bags, and, for healing purposes, in capsule and tincture forms. The usual dose for the tea is three cups a day. In tincture form, take one teaspoon up to three times a day. Otherwise, follow dose instructions on the bottle label.

SAFETY ISSUES: None.

### *Red Clover* (Trifolium pratense)

Red (aka purple) clover has been in the natural healer's medicine bag since the Greeks and Romans. It is used for a wide variety of complaints, from eczema to coughs. It also contains a form of vitamin E that has been shown in animal studies to prevent the formation of breast tumors.

DOSE: Take one cup of the tea three times a day or ½ to 1½ teaspoons of the fluid extract three times a day.

SAFETY ISSUES: None.

### *Sarsaparilla* (Smilax officinalis)

Clinical reports indicate that sarsaparilla root and berries tone the sex organs and glands and increase sex drive and energy. Sarsaparilla is an excellent tonic herb that can be taken for weeks or months in order to restore strength and vitality to the sex organs and glands. Traditional American herbalists recommend sarsaparilla tonics in the spring and fall to nurture sexual function and increase energy.

DOSE: You can take this herb in tea, capsule, or extract form as a general daily tonic, for months at a time. Take ten drops of extract or one capsule in the morning and evening after meals. You can also drink three cups of tea a day.

SAFETY ISSUES: Sarsaparilla hardly has any side effects. The sole possibility is a rise in blood pressure, which can easily be countered by the vitamin C and electrolytes contained in a single glass of orange juice.

### *Saw palmetto* (Serenoa repens)

Saw palmetto is a small palm tree native to the West Indies and the Atlantic coast from South Carolina to Florida. Native

Americans used saw palmetto berries to treat genitourinary tract disturbances and as a tonic to nutritionally support the entire body. It was also used to increase sperm production and to soothe irritated mucous membranes, particularly those of the genitourinary tract and prostate gland. Women used it to correct disorders of the mammary glands, and traditional healers claim that long-term use causes the breasts to enlarge. Many herbalists consider saw palmetto to be a long-term aphrodisiac, and it is currently used to prevent and relieve inflammation and swelling of the prostate.

*DOSE:* Take one 80 to 200 mg capsule after each meal. Make sure the capsule is standardized to give 85 to 95 percent of fatty acid sterols. The key to getting enough saw palmetto is standardization. Over twenty double-blind, placebo-controlled studies have demonstrated that the fat-soluble extract of the berries standardized to contain 85 to 95 percent fatty acids and sterols is effective in relieving all of the major symptoms of BPH. It is particularly effective when used in conjunction with pygeum.

The bark from Pygeum *(Pygeum africanum)*, an evergreen tree native to Africa, is used in combination with palm oil or milk by traditional African healers in order to treat urinary tract disorders. Western natural health-care providers prize pygeum for its powerful action on the prostate, which is accomplished mainly through normalizing hormone output and by preventing accumulation of cholesterol in the prostate.

*SAFETY ISSUES:* None.

## *Squaw Vine* (Mitchella repens)

Though many herbalists recommend squaw vine tea or tincture to relieve bloat and as a general female tonic and cleanser, squaw vine is best reserved for external uses, as it has a high wax content that can clog the liver.

It makes an effective douche (use the standard infusion recipe, then cool) to cleanse the vaginal area of common vaginitis. Cycles of urinary tract infections can be broken by douching with squaw vine tea at the first hint of discomfort. Urinary tract infections are commonly caused by an overabundance of E coli bacteria, which thrives in the rectum. UTIs, as these infections are commonly known, can also signal a persistent vaginitis.

*DOSE:* Use a weak tea to douche.

*SAFETY ISSUES:* None.

### *Valerian Root* (Valeriana officinalis)

Though valerian root has been used throughout Western history for everything from stomach discomfort and migraines to the plague, its primary effect is sedative because it relaxes muscles and nerves. Some herbalists recommend stuffing your pillow with this root to promote a peaceful night's sleep or the relaxed state of mind that is most conducive to great sex.

*DOSE:* Valerian root can be taken as a tea or by capsule or tincture. The usual dose is two capsules, one cup of the tea, or ten to fifteen drops of the tincture, taken a half hour before bedtime. Another option is to take a long, warm bath infused with fifteen to twenty drops of valerian decoction or oil.

*SAFETY ISSUES:* Valerian is approved by the United States Food and Drug Administration, but there is some question about the safety of valerian's active ingredients in large doses.

## ANCIENT COMPOUND TONIC REMEDIES

Compound tonic remedies mix a group of herbs together so that their synergistic effect balances and stimulates particular body systems and increases tone. Tonics make wonderful preventative treatments that enhance vitality and well-being. But they can also be effective once disease or dysfunction has set in.

If you are susceptible to a weakness in the sex organs and glands or are over forty, it's a good idea to make a tonic formula part of your daily routine. Bringing the body systems into balance usually takes a few weeks, and the effects should last for several months.

For example, most men over fifty suffer some problem with their prostate gland. Start taking the male tonic herbs pygeum and saw palmetto every day at age forty for one of the most effective ways to cut down on this risk (along with eating any of the seeds listed in chapter 1, for their zinc content). In recent years a few companies have come out with tinctures and capsules that contain both these herbs plus zinc.

Tonics can also be beneficial before forty. Modern women often combine the demands of full-time careers with full-time family care. They would be wise to take tonics that promote strength, energy, sexual function, and a hardy, balanced nervous system for at least two weeks out of every month or—with caution and only with the approval of your doctor—during pregnancy.

One of the oldest and most powerfully effective Chinese herbal compound tonics is Ten Significant Tonic Decoction (Chinese name: *Shi-quan-da-bu-tang*), which dates back to A.D. 1,200. It includes many herbal ingredients that are still popular today, particularly licorice, rehmannia, panax ginseng, and astragalus, and was specifically formulated to enhance sexual vitality. Since making this tonic yourself is difficult, purchase a commercial preparation. If you do not live near a Chinese herbal pharmacy, you can order this tonic from any one of several mail-order companies.

Essiac, another compound tonic, draws on the healing wisdom of various Native North American tribes. It too contains herbs that are still popular today: burdock, slippery elm, sheep sorrel, and turkey rhubarb. Essiac is too complex to make on your own, but it is also available at some health food stores and through mail-order companies.

## Homemade Tonic Recipes

Many tonic formulations—those that follow ancient recipes or new compounds developed by modern-day herbal scientists—are readily available at your health food store or by mail order.

The following list offers a selection of easy-to-make turn-on tonics. Any one of them can be taken safely over the long term to protect your sexual health, kindle your sexual desire, and enhance your lovemaking experience.

### TONICS FOR WOMEN

#### *Chinese Female-Strengthening Tonic*

1 cup whiskey
1 cup honey
1 cup lemon juice

Combine the ingredients and stir until the honey dissolves. Put the mixture in a glass jar and store in a cool, dry place. It is not necessary to refrigerate. Shake the jar well before each use. This tonic lasts several months—thanks to the whiskey—and the older it gets, the better it works.

*DOSE:* Take one to two tablespoons daily.

*SAFETY ISSUES:* Do not take during a menstrual period or when pregnant.

### *Chinese Chicken Soup*

For this simple recipe, you need whole, fresh dong quai, which can be purchased in Chinese markets and herb stores.

Place one to two heads of the herb (about one inch in size) in chicken broth or soup and season as desired. Simmer in a slow cooker for approximately three to five hours.

After drinking this soup regularly for a month or two, you will notice a marked increase in your overall strength and sexual function.

*DOSE:* Drink freely.

*SAFETY ISSUES:* None.

### *Fennel-Licorice Sex Tonic*

Simmer two teaspoons of slightly crushed fennel seeds and one ounce of minced licorice root in one pint of water for twenty minutes. Let stand until cool. Strain.

*DOSE:* Take two tablespoons twice a day.

*SAFETY ISSUES:* None.

## TONICS FOR MEN

### *Pygeum and Saw Palmetto Tea*

Although a tincture is stronger, you can make a decoction that uses equal parts of these two herbs by following the standard recipe for decoctions.

### HERBAL MENSTRUAL CRAMP RELIEF

St. John's wort, taken in extract form, 300 mg once or twice daily, or dong quai, one to two 500 mg capsules three times a day, are helpful.

You can also mix a few drops of marjoram, lavender, and chamomile essential oils into a massage oil made from a cold-pressed vegetable oil such as sunflower or olive oil. Rub on your belly to relieve menstrual cramps.

*DOSE:* Drink three to four cups a day.
*SAFETY ISSUES:* None.

### *American Indian Ginseng Combination Tea*

Mix together one tablespoon each of powdered ginseng root, parsley root, and wild columbine. Pour 1½ pints of boiling water over the herb mixture. Cover and steep for ten to fifteen minutes. Strain.

*DOSE:* Drink one cup three times a day, or as needed.
*SAFETY ISSUES:* None.

## UNISEX TONIC RECIPES

### *Hops-Citrus Sex Tonic*

Simmer the peel of two lemons and one orange in one quart of water for twenty minutes. Add three tablespoons of dried hops and simmer for three minutes. Remove from the heat and stir in honey to taste. Cover and cool to lukewarm. Add three tablespoons of lecithin, mixing well.

*DOSE:* Take half a cup three or four times a day.
*SAFETY ISSUES:* None.

### *Gypsy Love Tea*

Mix together one ounce each of hops, alfalfa, agrimony, and centaury. Add one quarter of water and bring to a boil. Cover and simmer for fifteen minutes. Remove from the heat, strain, and cool.

*DOSE:* Take half a cup before meals three times a day.

*SAFETY ISSUES:* None.

### *American Indian Libido Gruel*

Bring two tablespoons of unrefined oatmeal (which tones the sex glands and organs), half a cup of raisins, and one quart of water to a boil. Cover and simmer for forty-five minutes. Remove from the heat and strain. Add honey to taste. Cool and add half a teaspoon of lemon juice.

*DOSE:* Take one cup as needed.

*SAFETY ISSUES:* None.

### *Fenugreek Seed with Honey*

This valuable seed is rich in vitamin A, a lack of which is often found in men suffering from impotency. Since these seeds contain a chemical that acts as a sex hormone in frogs and speeds up flower production in plants, many cultures also believe that these seeds cure male impotence and lack of desire in females. You can brew the tea (see p. 37) or try these tasty honey treats.

Grind the seeds into a powder. (Use a coffee grinder or a blender at high speed or try an old-fashioned mortar and pestle.) Mix with an equal part of honey.

*DOSE:* Take by the tablespoonful as often as desired.

*SAFETY ISSUES:* None.

### *Sesame Combination Treat*

This delicious dessert paste is a quick energy tonic and hormone booster. Simmer three tablespoons of sesame seed, one ounce of licorice root, and a quarter pound of pitted, minced dates in two quarts of water until the liquid is reduced to one quart. Remove from the heat and add one cup of honey, stirring well until the mixture is well blended.

*DOSE:* Take two tablespoons three or four times a day, or as needed.

*SAFETY ISSUES:* None.

# 3

# THE SUPPLEMENT CONNECTION

Like the renewed interest in herbology, today's heightened focus on supplements results, in part, from a general disenchantment with conventional medicine. Increasingly, supplements are being used to help prevent disease and dysfunction and to heal many sex-related problems. When used correctly, supplements can balance, tone, and strengthen your sex organs and glands. They also restore body chemicals that naturally dwindle with age, thereby increasing sexual eagerness and intensifying your lovemaking experience.

Ideally, you should meet your vitamin and mineral quota through diet rather than by taking supplements. Many of us believe that we are receiving all the vitamins, minerals, and other essential nutrients we need from our diets. Sadly, we are usually mistaken. We live in an era of huge industrial farms, where high production is the aim, often at the expense of nutritional content. Fruits, vegetables, and other foods are sprayed with harmful chemicals and grown in soil deficient in essential trace minerals and saturated in pesticides. Eating organically grown foods whenever possible, plus taking supplements, can make up for the deficiencies caused by these modern farming methods and overprocessing of foods.

Supplements can carry their own risks, however. Many vitamins and minerals are water-soluble—that is, they are not stored in the body's fatty tissues and therefore cannot build to toxic levels. But taking supplements, which are stored in the body's fatty tissues, can be hazardous, because they can build to toxic levels. And even those water-soluble nutrients can cause problems if they are taken in excessive amounts that tax the kidneys and bladder—

key components of the body's filtration system. Since the urinary and genital systems are related, your sexual function can be weakened in this way.

The right supplements in the right amounts will help to keep you strong and toned—inside and out—maintaining, even restoring sexual desire, along with energy and stamina. Of course, no single pill or capsule will turn you into a sex machine, but the right supplement program provides the nutrients you need to become more vital and turn your bedroom into a bower of bliss.

The subject of supplements can be daunting. With all the extravagant claims being made by thousands of supplement manufacturers, how can you know what you should take? Which are the real sex boosters? What really works? What's best for me? This chapter gives you guidelines to make the correct supplement choices for you.

## Multivitamin-Mineral Supplements

The greatest boost to your sex life can be a good multivitamin-mineral supplement. If you choose the right combinations, dose levels, and a reputable brand, you will keep your vitamin and mineral intake at optimum levels, and with minimum effort on your part. All you have to do is pop a few pills two to three times a day, usually right after your meals.

Some physicians and nutritionists claim that any multivitamin-mineral will do, that it doesn't matter whether or not a supplement is "natural." Natural health-care providers strongly disagree. Quality varies from manufacturer to manufacturer, and important guidelines should be kept in mind when choosing any vitamin or mineral supplement.

1. Buy hypoallergenic supplements. Many people are allergic or "sensitive" (a broader term that includes more subtle adverse reactions that conventional doctors often dismiss or overlook) to the binders and fillers used in many tablets. These include waxes, clays, and dyes. Look for a brand that is labeled "hypoallergenic," which means it is free of allergenic binders and fillers.

When it comes to multivitamin-mineral supplements, you do get what you pay for. As a general rule, the cheaper the supplement, the more allergenic it is.

2. Don't buy supplements labeled "time-release." These con-

tain clays that slow the absorption in your digestive tract. Even if you notice no adverse reactions at first, repeated exposure over time can cause you to become allergic to the clays.

3. Avoid one-a-day brands. They deliver excessively high levels of the supplement in one pill or capsule. It's better to space out your supplement intake over the day, taking one with each meal.

4. While many manufacturers make bogus claims that their supplement is "natural," a natural supplement should derive its nutrients from concentrated sources of foods, like beet or alfalfa. Read labels carefully.

5. Watch dose levels of particular vitamins. Fat-soluble vitamins—A, D, E, and K (aka menadiol)—are stored in the body. If taken to excess, these fat-soluble vitamins will build to toxic levels in your body and make you sick. Symptoms to watch out for include fatigue, nausea, headaches, low blood sugar, joint pain, and hair loss. Other vitamins, such as vitamin C, are water soluble. Since excess amounts are excreted by the kidneys, most experts claim that high levels of water-soluble vitamins are safe. But overdosing on vitamin C can cause abdominal cramps and diarrhea, as well as irritation of the urogenital system that can become chronic and be mistaken for a urinary tract infection. Check the amounts of each vitamin and mineral provided by the supplement against the recommended doses that follow and/or the recommendations from your natural health-care provider.

6. Look on the bottle label of your mineral supplements for the amino acids "aspartate," "picolinate," "malate," or "citrate." Experts estimate that as little as 10 percent of most mineral supplements are actually absorbed. A good supplement attaches its mineral components to the above amino acids in order to increase their absorbability. Avoid calcium carbonate, which is made from ground-up oyster shells and is very tough on the digestive system.

7. Never take a heavy-duty vitamin-mineral supplement on an empty stomach or with your morning coffee. This can cause cramps and nausea and inhibit the body's ability to absorb the nutrients effectively. Always take a supplement either in the middle of a meal or within twenty minutes of finishing a meal, unless otherwise directed.

8. Don't keep an open bottle of supplements over six to nine months. Keep supplement bottles in the refrigerator, especially if they contain fats or oils.

RECOMMENDED CONTENTS AND AMOUNTS FOR A MULTIVITAMIN-MINERAL SUPPLEMENT

| | |
|---|---|
| **VITAMINS** | |
| Vitamin A | 4,000–10,000 I.U. (international unit) |
| Vitamin D | 200–600 I.U. |
| Vitamin E | 100–600 I.U. |
| Vitamin C | 500–2,000 mg (milligrams) |
| Vitamin $B_1$ (thiamine) | 50–150 mg |
| Vitamin $B_2$ (riboflavin) | 10–30 mg |
| Vitamin $B_3$ (niacin) | 100–300 mg |
| Vitamin $B_5$ (pantothenic acid) | 80–120 mg |
| Vitamin $B_6$ | 100–200 mg |
| Vitamin $B_{12}$ | 10–100 mg |
| Vitamin K | 70–100 mcg (micrograms) |
| **MINERALS** | |
| Calcium | 300–800 mg |
| Chromium | 50–200 mcg |
| Copper | 2–3 mg |
| Zinc | 15–40 mg* |
| Folic acid | 400–800 mcg |
| Iodine | 150–225 mcg |
| Iron | 18 mg |
| Magnesium | 300–800 mg |
| Manganese | 1–10 mg |
| Molybdenum | 15–500 mcg |
| Potassium | 90–100 mcg |
| Selenium | 50–200 mcg |

*Older men can use as much as 60 mg a day.

## VITAMINS AND MINERALS THAT ENHANCE SEXUAL VITALITY

When establishing a multivitamin-mineral program tailored to your individual needs, you should be aware of the following vitamins, minerals, and other essential nutrients that are key to optimum sexual functioning. During times of stress or illness and as we age, we often need higher levels of some nutrients.

### *Vitamin A*

The usual recommended vitamin A supplement is 25,000 I.U. of betacarotene, depending on how well your body converts vegetable and fruit sources of carotenoids in vitamin A. A daily teaspoonful of cod liver oil or betacarotene tablets, both of which are high in vitamin A, nutritionally supports sexual function. Recent studies confirm that betacarotene is a safer way of supplementing vitamin A, because excess levels are less likely to build to toxic levels in the body.

If you have an infection, you can go as high as 100,000 I.U. of betacarotene, but return to the 25,000 I.U. dose once the infection subsides. Make sure that you're also taking at least 30 mg of zinc to help your body convert the betacarotene into vitamin A.

### *Vitamin E*

The standard recommended dose of vitamin E is 200 I.U. of natural mixed tocoherols per day in capsule or tablet form. The natural form is used more effectively by the body than the synthetic d-alpha tocopherols. If your sexual desire is low, have your vitamin E blood levels checked. The normal adult tocopherol blood level is 0.5 mg per 100 ml (milliliter) of blood plasma. If you have less than this level, your body will reflect this lack in its poor sexual function. If this is the case, increase your dose by 200 to 400 I.U.

### *B Complex*

If you lack energy, have poor resistance to colds and flus, and suffer from low libido, check your doctor first to rule out any medical condition that could be causing your symptoms. Many people with this vague array of symptoms are given a clean bill of health by their doctor. Their health is not good, but the doctor can't assign the blame for their substandard condition to any specific disease or dysfunction. In such cases, B vitamins can restore energy and sexual desire.

One common cause of waning sexual desire is hypothyroidism, or an underactive thyroid, which is also linked to chronic fatigue and hair loss. If this is your problem, see your doctor and eat foods high in vitamin $B_1$ (see chapter 1) and take 150 mg of $B_1$ daily in supplement form to perk up your lagging libido.

In cases of extreme chronic fatigue, you can take 50 mg three times a day. Another good solution is to take 100 mg of vitamin $B_2$ (riboflavin), along with 200 mg of vitamin $B_3$ (niacin) and 500 mg of pantothenic acid. Niacin causes a temporary flush of the skin, accompanied by a sensation of heat in the entire body. Some people love it, but others find the sensation disturbing and uncomfortable.

An alternative is taking 200 mg of niacinamide, another type of $B_3$. This also has a sedative effect on jangled nerves, because it raises your levels of the feel-good hormone, serotonin. One gram of niacinamide before bedtime can put you in the mood for love and counter insomnia. Before getting a prescription for a pharmaceutical antidepressant, try a program that combines the herb St. John's wort along with niacinamide.

B complex relies on magnesium to be activated, so make sure your magnesium intake is sufficient. Standard daily dose of a B vitamin complex supplement is 50 mg per day.

### *Vitamin C*

Without this valuable antioxidant, sperm clump together and lose their mobility. Take 1 to 3,000 mg of vitamin C for optimum maintenance of the sex glands and organs in both sexes; it also helps make skin satin smooth and caressable. The newest facial creams contain high levels of vitamin C to help aging skins speed up collagen repair, thus improving elasticity and countering wrinkles and sagging.

You can derive up to 200 mg of vitamin C a day from a well-balanced diet that includes C-rich foods like citrus fruits. But unless you eat large amounts of citrus and dark green leafy vegetables every day, you would benefit from supplements of vitamin C tablets, powder, or capsules.

Establish your optimum vitamin C supplement level by increasing your dosage incrementally. When you reach a dosage that gives you diarrhea and/or any other gastrointestinal discomfort, cut down the dosage until you no longer experience any symptoms. Another sign that you are taking too much vitamin C

## VITAMIN C SENSITIVITY

Cutting-edge research being conducted by Dr. Devi Nambudripad of The Pain Clinic, located in Buena Park, California, suggests that these high levels of intravenous vitamin C as well as overly high doses of any supplement, can actually create a condition of oversensitivity that can cause many "mysterious" yet persistent inflammatory conditions, particularly chronic inflammation of the urogenital and digestive tracts. Sensitivity to vitamin C (as well as to any vitamin, mineral, or nutrient) can aggravate, rather than relieve, symptoms of chronic fatigue and sexual malaise.

While there is no scientifically validated test for this sensitivity, Dr. Nambudripad and other doctors trained in her desensitization technique, N.A.E.T. (Nambudripad Allergy Elimination Technique), have much clinical evidence and preliminary study results to support their claims. To determine the presence of a sensitivity, they use a technique from kinesiology called "muscle testing," which is practiced by many alternative doctors, chiropractors, and other holistic health-care providers.

If your doctor recommends high doses of vitamin C as part of your rejuvenation program, and you do not experience relief after a week or so of treatment, discuss stopping the treatment and exploring other options.

is if you experience irritation when urinating. Again, cut back your dose to a more comfortable level.

Many alternative medical doctors use high doses of vitamin C to treat a variety of diseases and dysfunction, particularly for those generalized and vague complaints of low energy and malaise that elude conventional diagnosis, and for chronic infections. They often administer C in combination with other vitamins and minerals through an intravenous solution to boost immunity and energy. Intravenous doses range from twenty to forty grams at a time, which runs as high as six hundred times the U.S. Recommended Daily Allowance of 45 mg of vitamin C a day.

### *Magnesium*

Magnesium is a great muscle relaxant that gives you the suppleness you need for intense, blockbuster orgasms (which are, after all, a series of muscular contractions and relaxations). Always take magnesium with calcium, in a ratio of two parts calcium to one part magnesium. Most supplements already come in that ratio, and it's an especially good idea to find a supplement that combines calcium with magnesium as well as phosphorus, in the ratio described in chapter 1.

Magnesium's beneficial effects on the muscles also make it a good remedy to prevent and relieve PMS and menstrual cramps. If you suffer chronically from either or both of these problems, take an extra 100 mg of magnesium glyconate (the most absorbable form) every two hours at the first sign of cramps and make sure you are getting adequate levels of this important mineral throughout the month. Standard dose is a supplement that contains 1,000 mg of calcium and 500 mg of magnesium, taken at bedtime.

### *Zinc*

Found in high concentrations in seminal fluid, zinc helps men achieve and maintain hard erections. Zinc is also essential to female sexual function. Be careful not to exceed your optimum level, as too much zinc adversely affects your absorption of iron, calcium, and copper. Your smartest move would be not to supplement zinc unless your doctor or alternative health-care provider has checked your zinc blood levels and found them lacking.

---

### MENSTRUAL CRAMP COMBO

Magnesium taken in a dose of 400 to 600 mg, in combination with 50 mg of vitamin $B_6$, eases uterine muscle spasms and helps balance sex hormone function. If your multivitamin-mineral supplement does not deliver these dosage levels, take extra supplements of magnesium and $B_6$. This supplement combination is also effective against PMS, which is thought by many experts to be caused by a disturbance in sex hormone balance, specifically by an excess level of estrogen. At the onset of cramps, also take an additional 100 mg of magnesium glyconate, a highly absorbable form of magnesium.

---

However, the body does not absorb zinc well, especially after age fifty, so zinc supplements in mature men and women are usually a good idea. Many studies suggest that zinc can prevent the all-too-common condition affecting men over fifty, enlargement and/or inflammation of the prostate gland (BPH).

The recommended dose for older men and women is 60 mg a day, divided into three doses of 20 mg each, but, again, determine your optimum dosage on the basis of blood levels.

## OTHER IMPORTANT SEX SUPPLEMENTS

### *Gamma-Linolenic Acid (GLA)*

The group of oils called essential fatty acids lubricate the sex glands of men and women, keeping them young and vital and pumping out the hormones that keep sexual desire and function at optimum levels. GLAs also help prevent many sex gland–related ailments. Take one to two tablespoons per day of cold-pressed flaxseed oil either alone or drizzled on your vegetables. Another option, especially after age fifty, is a mixed EFA complex capsule that gives you a balance of Omega 3s, 6s, and 9s. Take one capsule in the morning and one in the evening. All brands contain from 500 to 1,000 mg per capsule.

### *Bee Pollen*

Bee pollen, available in loose and capsule form, has been shown in studies to prevent menopausal complaints, nervous conditions, and ensure peak sexual function.

DOSE: If you decide to use bee pollen be careful, as it is highly allergenic. Use only the loose grains in order to avoid any allergic reaction. Start out with one grain of pollen with each meal. Add one grain per meal every day, until you reach a total dose of one teaspoon per day.

SAFETY ISSUES: See above.

### *Glutathione*

Glutathione is a powerful anti-oxidant, as effective, though not as popular, as vitamins C, E, and beta-carotene. Boosting blood

## ☙ ANTI-PMS SUPPLEMENT COMBO

To halt the mood swings associated with PMS, take evening primrose oil, a GLA, along with extra $B_6$. Recommended dose is one gram three times a day. Though some natural health-care providers recommend the less expensive flaxseed oil, it is thought by others to be less easily absorbed by the body.

$B_6$ helps break down estrogen, which can build to excessive levels and cause PMS. Take either 200 mg daily of $B_6$ or 50 mg of the activated form, P5P. $B_6$ also relieves water retention and breast tenderness before and during menstrual periods.

Environmental pollutants can aggravate PMS, so it's also a good idea to take supplements that will help your body defend itself against these toxins. Make sure to take your multivitamin-mineral, along with 1,000 mg of vitamin C and 400 mg of vitamin E every day.

## ☙ CHRONIC PELVIC INFLAMMATION REMEDY

A combined dose of vitamin E and flaxseed oil can help prevent inflammation, including the inflammation accompanying menstrual cramps, as well as interrupt chronic inflammatory conditions. Take one tablespoon of flaxseed oil and 400 I.U. of vitamin E every day. When cramping occurs, try taking 3,000 I.U. of bromelain, a natural enzyme with anti-inflammatory properties that is readily available in health food stores, twice a day, between meals.

levels of glutathione gives greater vitality and sexual energy. It also detoxifies the body naturally from environmental and bodily toxins that accumulate in the fatty deposits cushioning and protecting your sex organs and glands. This internal pollution blocks healthy sexual function, desire, and capacity for enjoyment and can eventually cause sex-organ or gland-related disease.

*DOSE:* Glutathione is found in fresh, unprocessed pork, veal, chicken, and beef, as well as in fresh whole fruits and vegetables—not juices—but since it is relatively insoluble, the body doesn't absorb glutathione well from the digestive tract. Therefore, it's best to take glutathione supplements in high doses. The standard dose is 100 to 500 mg per day. Men and women over forty can take as much as 1,000 to 3,000 mg per day.

Another way to increase glutathione blood levels is by taking at least 3,000 mg of vitamin C, which will act synergistically with 4,000 mg of L-glutamine per day—in divided doses.

***SAFETY ISSUES:*** None.

# 4

# THE EXERCISE CONNECTION

Along with renewed interest in diet, healing herbs, and supplements, many people are turning to exercise in order to increase their sexual health and pleasure, even to various traditional Eastern exercises such as yoga and Taoist postures. Interest is also building in Eastern medical modalities, like acupressure and acupuncture, because they strengthen and heal by stimulating the body's own healing powers. Western bodywork and therapeutic touch therapies that stem from these Eastern practices, such as Rolfing and the Alexander Technique, also aim to prevent health problems—particularly those inhibiting full sexual response and function—by strengthening the patient, physically and mentally.

Traditional Eastern healers and philosophers have understood the profound connection between physical exercise and sexuality for many centuries. In fact, certain types of yoga exercises from ancient India and virtually all the taoist exercises from ancient China were designed specifically to help their practitioners enjoy longer-lasting, more intense, and deeply satisfying lovemaking.

We in the modern West may be fitness fanatics, but it wasn't too long ago that women were discouraged from exercising because it would give them "masculine" musculature and because exercise was viewed as somehow improper for ladies. Though we've come a long way since then, we are only just beginning to understand the equation between exercise, health, and sex.

You are undoubtedly aware that exercise improves the appearance, tightening jiggly spots, smoothing out lumps and bumps, and generally making the body more toned, sleek, and sexually attractive. Some types of exercise commonly used to build muscles and improve strength and energy include weight, or strength, training; isometrics or resistance training; and calisthenics. And if you are a woman who is still afraid of developing muscles, keep in mind the truism that a strong man's ideal sex partner is a strong woman and that light weight training tones and defines muscles, without adding bulk.

## THE SEX BENEFITS OF REGULAR EXERCISE

Physical exercise can do even more for a sex life than build a hot, hard body and greater sexual energy. In fact, the relationship between sexuality and regular exercise, especially certain specific exercises, is far deeper and more extensive than most of us realize.

- After working out regularly for a few months, you naturally tune in to your body. You become more sensitive to its various workings—the stretch of your muscles, the blood pumping through your vessels—and you begin to take more physical enjoyment in this intricate miracle machine of yours. Exercising is no longer just a duty; it becomes your pleasure, a wonderfully sensual experience that carries over into your sex life.
- Better overall muscle tone helps your body enjoy the powerful contraction-release sensation of a full-body orgasm. (Orgasms result from muscles contracting and releasing in "waves.") Regular exercisers report more intense orgasmic sensations and more frequent orgasms. Improved pelvic muscle tone, in particular, helps you enjoy blockbuster orgasms.
- Increased overall strength makes you sexually fit in any position.
- Increased endurance helps you enjoy sexual encounters for as long as you wish.
- A more efficient metabolism. Making love burns about one hundred calories. If you're on top, you use up to 150 calories. That's the equivalent of walking twenty minutes at a brisk pace. You don't have to leave your bedroom, and you'll have a lot more fun.
- More sensitive and efficient body systems. Every body sys-

tem—nerves, lungs, heart, and blood vessels—all the parts involved in sexual arousal, lovemaking, and orgasm purr more smoothly.

- Better hormone production. Some experts theorize that regular exercisers may experience an increase in the male hormone testosterone, which is linked to sexual desire in both men and women.
- More endorphins. Other researchers note that immediately after a workout, blood levels of endorphins rise considerably. Endorphins are the body's feel-good hormones, natural painkillers that also promote a feeling of well-being, which is, of course, a sexual turn-on. While research has not proven that endorphins are connected directly to the libido, anecdotal evidence bears out this theory. Anyone who has experienced "runner's high" knows that exercise reduces anxiety and stress and banishes mild depression, putting you more in the mood for love.
- Better self-image. Yes, we all want to be loved for our "inner" selves. But keeping your body strong and fit boosts your self-image, at the same time it broadcasts to others that you take care of yourself and enjoy a healthy sense of pride. That psychological lift you get from the results of working out—your trim, shapely body—goes a long way toward combating any hang-ups you might have about your body image. Negative body image is a common obstacle to sexual enjoyment that can affect men, but seems to affect many more women. If you dislike your body, it's difficult to enjoy sex. And when you lack self-confidence, you're likely to project that negative self-image onto your partner. While the problem is mainly psychological and can be treated through guided visualizations and, if necessary, counseling, it doesn't hurt to hit the gym three times a week to build yourself a healthier, more attractive body.

Warning: Don't overdo it. Too much exercise or overly vigorous exercise can have the opposite effect, robbing you of stamina and energy, and dampening your libido instead of boosting it.

## SEX AS EXERCISE

The link between exercise and sex goes both ways, because sex itself is also a form of exercise. Psychoanalyst William Reich—who was deeply influenced by the traditional Eastern view of the reciprocal relationship between sex and health—advised his patients that an orgasm a day keeps the doctor away. Current research confirms the equation between an active sex life and robust health.

Sex can be aerobic—that is, as active as an aerobics session that elevates your blood-oxygen levels. If heavy lifting and other weight-bearing feats are also involved in a sexual encounter, it becomes anaerobic, producing results similar to the benefits of resistance training.

## The Health Benefits of Sex

- Slight elevation of "good" cholesterol, while your levels of "bad" cholesterol levels lower a bit.
- Deepens and quickens breathing, which pumps greater amounts of oxygen into your blood.
- Produces higher testosterone levels to increase libido in men and women.
- Floods your body with feel-good endorphins.
- Pumps up production of DHEA, the adrenal hormone currently touted as a miracle supplement for aging baby boomers. DHEA is thought to boost immunity, inhibit tumor growth, promote bone growth and density, elevate mood, and increase overall energy and sexual function. (See chapter 12 for more information on DHEA.)
- Drains the prostate gland of backed-up seminal fluids, which is of particular benefit to men over forty.
- Boosts estrogen production for women, especially menopausal women, which helps prevent heart disease, increase bone density, and keep vaginal tissues moist and supple.
- Helps to regulate menstrual periods and counter many PMS symptoms.

## Sexercises

What society may consider the so-called "perfect" body is not necessarily the most sexually fit body. We are not concerned here

## ❧ SEX FOR MENSTRUAL/PMS PROBLEMS

Studies prove that during masturbation women's pain thresholds rise. This suggests that sex—solo or with a partner, orgasmic or not—can ease menstrual cramps and chronic pain caused by such problems as arthritis and lower-back disorders. Experts theorize that this effect is explained, in part, by an overlap of the parts of the nervous system that control sensations of pain and pleasure. In other words, the feel-good endorphins released by sexual activity can give you enough pleasure to override your pain.

Taoist sex exercises and lovemaking practices are even more effective pain relievers than "ordinary" Western sex. See chapter 6 and chapter 9 for techniques that increase sexual desire as they strengthen and heal your pelvic organs and glands.

with ideal body proportions or with artificial body part enhancements that conform to fantasy media images of the sexy woman or man.

What we're talking about is regular exercise that improves overall health, stamina, and self-confidence, that helps you become stronger, more toned, and flexible, and puts you in touch with your body. Your added motivation for exercising is that all of these benefits prepare you for a more exciting and fulfilling sex life.

While any trainer at a gym can provide you with a good workout program, be sure to include the following specific "sexercises" to prime you for more intense, athletic, and pleasurable lovemaking. Always remember to inhale and exhale evenly while performing any exercise. Never hold your breath.

### *Pelvic Tilts*

This exercise increases your overall staying power by strengthening your back, abdominal muscles, and buttocks—all of which come into play during sexual intercourse. Strong abs and buttocks power the thrusts, bumps, and grinds of sexual intercourse.

1. Lie on your back, bend your knees, and place your feet flat on the floor, hip-width apart.
2. Squeeze your buttocks muscles tightly, at the same time contracting your abdominal muscles and pressing the small of your back into the floor.
3. Still pressing the small of your back into the floor, exhale as you push your hips toward the ceiling. Continue pushing your hips upward, maintaining the contraction in your butt and abs while keeping your upper back and feet on the ground. Hold at the highest point for a moment.
4. Slowly lower to the floor, unrolling your spine from the middle down to the bottom, then lowering your buttocks.

Start out with five repetitions and gradually work your way up to twenty. Rest for thirty seconds, then repeat.

### *Abdominal Crunches*

This exercise is the most effective and safest way to tone and strengthen your abdominals and lower back—essentials for active sex. Crunches also prevent and correct lower back pain and weakness often associated with debility in the sex organs and glands.

1. Lie on your back, knees bent, feet flat on the ground, in the same position as above.
2. Contract your buttocks, at the same time pressing your lower back into the floor.
3. Extend your arms along the sides of your body. Exhale as you raise your upper body, at the same time contracting your abs and pressing your lower spine into the floor. Gently take hold of the upper part of each inner thigh.

---

### BEST WESTERN EXERCISE SEX BOOSTERS

- Strength training: calisthenics, isometrics, weights
- Aerobic activity: running, cycling, aerobics classes, dancing, skiing and ski machines, jump-rope, mini-trampoline
- Sports: dancing, skating, gymnastics

---

4. Keeping your body in the same raised position—lower spine pressed into the floor, abdominals contracted—bend your elbows and lightly touch your hands to each ear.
5. Continue to press your lower spine against the floor and contract your abdominals for the count of six.
6. Relax back down to the floor.

Work your way up to twenty crunches twice a day.

## EXERCISING YOUR LOVE MUSCLE

The muscle most directly involved in the pleasures of sex and orgasm is the pubococcygeus, aka the PC or "love" muscle, located in the genital area. Traditional Eastern disciplines offer myriad exercises that tone and sensitize this muscle in order to stoke sexual desire and heat up lovemaking.

The West has only one exercise, although it is quite effective when practiced regularly—Kegels. "Kegeling" involves rhythmically contracting and relaxing the PC muscle, as if you were trying to stop the flow of urine. Although they are frequently written about in relation to women, Kegel exercises are also of great benefit to men.

### *The Benefits of Kegeling*

Like any other muscle exercised regularly, the PC muscle will become healthier and more toned and develop a richer blood and nerve supply. That translates into getting more sexually excited faster and enjoying more frequent, charged, and long-lasting orgasms.

A woman who can contract her PC muscle snugly around her partner's penis is a desirable love partner indeed! A man with a well-developed PC muscle can squeeze it in order to delay his orgasm. He can also squeeze to make his penis "jump" inside his partner—another sweet sensation for both of them.

### When to Kegel

Another great thing about Kegeling is that the exercises can be done anywhere, anytime, in front of anyone, and no one will be the wiser.

Establishing a regular Kegeling routine is up to you. You can "trick" yourself into a daily routine by linking Kegel sessions to other daily activities. Here are some suggestions:

- While showering or in the bath. (If women combine Kegeling with a fifteen minute soak in a salt water bath—using a half cup sea salt to a full tub of warm water—they are also cultivating an ideal vaginal environment.)
- While brushing and flossing. (The advantage of linking these two chores is that most of us do not clean our teeth long enough. This helps you to do both beneficial activities longer. It's also a good exercise in coordination—like patting your head and rubbing your tummy at the same time.)
- Before or after every meal.
- While you're waiting for a traffic light to change, or to pay a bridge or tunnel toll.
- While watching the television news.
- While on hold during a phone call.
- Standing in line at the bank, movie, or supermarket.

### How Often to Kegel

Ideally, Kegeling should be done three times a day, but do not assign yourself such an overly ambitious program that you can't follow it. You could become discouraged and stop Kegeling altogether.

After a month or two of regular practice, you should feel a marked increase in control over your urine stream and, more important, an increase in sexual pleasure.

### How to Kegel

There are different types of Kegel exercises. For best results, include each type in every session.

Before you start Kegeling, first practice stopping and starting the flow of urine until you become familiar with your PC muscle and gain some control over it.

#### PUMPS

Squeeze the PC muscle, hold for three seconds, then relax for three seconds. Repeat as many times as you can, working up to thirty 3-second squeezes at a time.

#### PULSES

Squeeze and relax the PC muscle quickly, in a fluttering motion. Start slowly at first, aiming for regular contractions rather than speed. Over time, you'll be able to do this at a faster, even pace.

#### BEAR-DOWNS

This variation also tones your lower abs. It's done by adding a gentle bearing down motion to your contractions-relaxations, as if you're having a bowel movement. Hold and release for three seconds at a time, working up to thirty sets. Don't be too forceful; the operative word is "gentle."

### *A Sample Kegeling Session*

Exhale as you give a short squeeze. Squeeze the PC muscle and anal sphincter fifteen to twenty times at approximately one squeeze per second. Make sure that your buttocks muscles are not contracting too; it's important to isolate and work only the PC muscle and anal sphincter. Gradually build up to two sets of seventy-five 1-second squeezes per day.

Squeeze the PC muscle and anal sphincter for a count of three. Relax for three counts. Work up to contracting for ten seconds, and relaxing for ten seconds. Start with two sets of twenty 3-second squeezes each and build up to seventy-five 10-second squeezes.

When you become practiced and toned, add very gentle bear-downs. After releasing the contraction, push down and out gently with your PC muscle and anal sphincter, as if you were having a bowel movement. Start with two sets of twenty bear-downs, and build up to seventy-five bear-downs.

You can work up to three hundred Kegel repetitions a day, combining short and long squeezes and bear-downs.

After two months of three hundred Kegel squeezes daily, you will have a strong, well-developed PC muscle. You can maintain that tone, flexibility, and control by doing only 150 repetitions several times a week.

## Sex Stretches

A pliant spine and flexible muscles are the key to eternal youth and a lifetime of great sex. A flexible lower spine is particularly essential because it helps you enjoy full pelvic mobility and sensation. If your spine and pelvis are rigid and tight, it is impossible to make the natural thrusting, bumping, grinding, and circular "winding" movements that heat up sexual intercourse and inevitably lead to powerful, long-lasting orgasms that extend to every cell of the body.

In fact, one reason why so many American women cannot orgasm from intercourse and so many men are not fulfilling their orgasmic potential is that they are like blocks of wood from the chest to the knees. In other words, a perfectly sculpted body may conform to popular notions of ideal male and female sex appeal, but it could be the barrier between that person and true sexual enjoyment. Those firm muscles may be overly tight, frozen in chronic contractions that impair deep breathing, numb sensation, and block sexual enjoyment.

Many of us suffer from this muscular rigidity. We are not flexible or free enough to breathe deeply and articulate the pelvic, abdominal, and spinal movements that are key to profound sexual feeling and enjoyment.

This chapter and later chapters give you the information you need to release that tight musculature so that you can "wind your waistline," as Caribbean people term it; that is, swivel, bump, and grind your hips and pelvis. The following exercises make for a good beginning.

### *Basic Body Stretch*

If you've ever seen a cat stretch, you know how wonderfully sensuous stretching can be. You can actually feel your body release tension; you automatically inhale more deeply, oxygenate your blood more thoroughly, and release toxins. A stretched-out, limber body is a sexually fit body, and no workout is complete without stretching every part, to keep muscles from shortening and losing their flexibility.

If you add a nice loud sigh to your exhalations, you'll discover that the benefits are even greater: your body becomes even more relaxed, your capacity to stretch increases, and your mind feels more at ease.

The following are great stretches to do before and/or after your exercise routine or simply on their own.

1. Lie on your back, arms comfortably extended over your head and a little out to the sides, legs extended and pointing slightly to each side.

---

### ❧ DANCING AND SEX

The link between dancing and sex is obvious. Alone or with a partner, dancing freely—moving wherever the music and your spirit take you—is a tremendously liberating and sensual experience. Put your favorite music on the stereo and let loose. You will probably laugh—maybe even feel a bit embarrassed at first. Don't let that stop you. Dance every day to recharge your energy and free your soul. Belly or Middle Eastern dancing, all African dancing, East Indian dancing, reggae dancing from Jamaica, and soca and calypso dancing from Trinidad and Tobago are particularly beneficial to your sex life because they help make your torso more mobile.

Take classes, or buy a videotape and dance along. Or go to an African, Middle Eastern, Indian, or Caribbean dance club. Have fun! Learning to "wind your wasitline"—that is, recovering your natural flexibility—prepares you for more pleasurable sexual intercourse.

---

2. Push your heels forward, at the same time that you press your lower spine against the floor.
3. Press and release your spine a few times to limber it up.
4. Now that your lower spine has enjoyed a little stretch, press it against the floor again, at the same time stretching your arms away from your head and your legs in the opposite direction, extending your heels. Be sure to keep all four limbs on the floor. Inhale as you stretch and feel your muscles release with each exhalation.

A terrific additional variation is to curve both arms and legs to the right side and then the left—making sure to keep the back pressed into the floor. This helps release the sides of the torso and gives the limbs an even greater stretch.

### *Sitting Forward Stretch*

This is another good stretch to keep your spine flexible.

1. Sit comfortably on the floor, legs extended straight in front of you, a little less than hip-width apart.
2. Use your hands to lift your buttocks off the floor and make sure that you're seated forward on your hips and your spine is straight.
3. Bending from the hip joints rather than your back, lean forward, keeping the back straight. At the same time, extend your heels forward to maximize the stretch. Think of bringing the lower abdomen closer to the thighs.

Don't worry about how far you bend. Hold and take ten slow, deep breaths. You should feel the stretch in the back of the calves and hamstrings.

### *Backbend Stretch*

This exercise stretches and loosens the muscles all along the front of your body. Do not do this if you have chronic lower back problems. Instead, do the abdominal stretching and strengthening exercises described in the chapter that follows this one.

1. Sit on a mat or cushion placed on the floor, buttocks on

heels, thighs together, knees bent, and lower legs tucked under your thighs.

2. Place your hands on the floor and behind your hips to support you.

3. Squeezing the buttocks tightly and pushing the hips forward, arch the upper body back slightly, stretching the front of the thighs and the entire trunk.

4. Stretch your chin up and slightly back, but do not let your head drop back all the way as this can damage the neck vertebra.

5. Hold the stretch as you inhale and exhale, slowly and evenly, at least ten times, feeling your body let go with each long exhalation.

# YOGA

"Yoga" means the union of body and mind through breath. This venerable Eastern discipline developed in India three to five thousand years ago and has influenced many of the newer holistic Western exercise and bodywork systems described later in this chapter.

Tantric yoga, which is covered in chapter 5, includes many powerful exercises that were designed specifically to enhance sexual energy and pleasure.

## HATHA YOGA

Hatha yoga, the form with which Westerners are most familiar, focuses on energizing, toning, and making the body more flexible. It consists of physical postures and breathing exercises that enhance overall physical health. But that doesn't make their benefits to sexuality any less potent. Establishing a regular yoga practice as part of your daily or weekly routine is one of the most effective ways you can secure good health and increase your sexual passion and pleasure.

The main difference between yoga and Western exercise is that yoga emphasizes inner, along with outer, health. The breath is also used to promote a greater sense of well-being and self-awareness and to facilitate performing the various postures. Unlike

Western exercises, which can exhaust you, yoga never causes you to lose energy. Instead, you gain vitality and a more balanced and even energy. Yoga improves endurance and flexibility and gives a stronger, more flexible spine and joints. It also calms the mind and spirit, making both body and mind more supple and sensual—ready and primed for good sex.

Although yoga teachers recommend practicing yoga at least one hour several times a week, there are simple yoga postures, or "asanas," you can do almost anywhere and in very little time.

If possible, yoga should be practiced in loose clothing and at least two hours after a meal. However, a few yoga stretches or breaths, practiced anywhere, are better than not doing them at all. Yoga is not a competitive sport but a wonderful gift you can give yourself. Do the yoga postures at your own pace, never forcing your body into any position it's not ready for. While yoga classes are strongly recommended so that you can be monitored and corrected, these easy and simple postures can be done almost anywhere.

## BASIC EASTERN BREATH

Most of us in the West are shallow breathers who use only one-seventh to one-third of our lung capacity, robbing ourselves not only of oxygen, but of the life-force energy we need for good health and passionate sex. Few of us breathe deeply enough to fully energize and sensitize our pelvic areas—the center of our sexuality. When we fill the pelvic girdle with fresh oxygen, we bring energy, warmth, and life to the sex organs and glands. Virtually all Eastern disciplines begin with the breath because it carries into and out of the body the universal energy, or "chi," that animates us and connects us to the greater whole. The Basic Eastern Breath is common to all Eastern disciplines.

Breath control means control of your energy, and its benefits are limitless. It helps to visualize your pelvis as a balloon that inflates with air on inhalation, then deflates on exhalation. This deep breathing pattern will "wake up" sexual feelings and energize and strengthen all the organs and glands.

For most Eastern breathing exercises, breathe in and out through the nostrils only, unless otherwise instructed.

1. Lie on your back with knees bent, feet about hip-width apart and planted on the floor. Make sure the small of the back is relaxed against the floor. You may want to place a rolled-up pillow or towel under your knees to help the abdomen and back relax completely.

2. Place the right hand gently on your lower abdomen and the left on your chest. Inhale, slowly, evenly, and deeply, so that the right hand rises. The left hand should stay still. As you exhale, the right hand should lower.

3. Close your eyes to help you tune into your breath and become aware of how it is filling and energizing your body.

4. Take several long, slow, deep breaths, trying to expand your abdomen a little more with each inhalation. Never force or hold your breath.

5. Now imagine that each inhalation is filling your entire torso. The top is your neck and the bottom is the perineum (the area between the anus and ureter—the opening of the urinary tract). The sides include the circumference of the rib cage, the stomach, back, and sides.

6. Inhale, first filling the bottom, then the top, and finally the entire circumference. Feel your rib cage expand as you inhale. Feel your genital area expand with energy and a deliciously alive sensation. Allow the space between the shoulder blades to relax open.

7. As you continue taking long inhalations and exhalations, allow your breath to travel into the legs and arms, filling your limbs with vital energy all the way down to the tips of the fingers and toes.

This breath may feel awkward at first, but after you've practiced it regularly for a while, it will become easy, familiar, and automatic.

Great times to practice are in the morning, before you get out of bed and start your day, and at night, before you drop off to sleep. The Basic Eastern Breath is a wonderful way to shed tensions at the end of the day. It also eases insomnia.

Once you are comfortable with this breathing exercise while lying down, practice it in a sitting position, always making sure that the abdomen is moving out with each inhalation and in with each exhalation, and that the chest stays still. You can use the breath when you're stuck in traffic, on line, or any time you find yourself in a boring or stressful situation.

This is the basic breath you will use in every yoga asana, as well as in the taoist exercises that follow.

### *Alternate Nostril Breathing*

This breathing exercise calms the mind, purifies and energizes the entire body, and makes you aware of the life force that flows throughout your body. You deliberately slow and balance the breath in order to destress the heart and central nervous system and to steady the metabolism.

Find a quiet place to be alone, such as your office or a bathroom. Sit with your back straight so that the lungs have maximum room to expand. This is also a great practice for morning or night, and it is an especially effective way to mark the transition between work and home, so you feel more relaxed and ready to enjoy a sensual evening with your partner.

1. Exhale completely, contracting and drawing in the abdominal muscles to force air from your lungs.
2. Close the right nostril with the right thumb, then slowly inhale through the left nostril. Do not overinflate your lungs.
3. When they are filled to comfortable capacity, also close the left nostril, using the fourth and fifth fingers and folding the index and middle fingers into the palm to keep them out of the way.
4. When you have filled your lungs and closed off both nostrils, hold the breath inside the lungs as long as possible without discomfort.

   When you first start to practice, the period of retention will not be long, but it will increase as you proceed.
5. As soon as you feel any discomfort, open the right nostril and, keeping the left one closed with the fourth and fifth fingers, slowly exhale.

These three phases—exhalation, inhalation, and block-switch—constitute a round (which always begins and ends on an exhalation), that is, one complete cycle.

If you're a first timer, try six to ten rounds for three to five minutes. Let the breath flow silently, a sign that it's not being forced. After a few rounds, exhale and inhale to the count of four. As you gain control, make your exhalations twice as long as your inhalations, and gradually increase the total number of rounds to twenty or more.

If you have the time, you can practice this exercise several times a day. Otherwise, once a day, or whenever you feel stressed, is enough.

## HATHA YOGA POSTURES (ASANAS)

These poses can be done together as a regular yoga session or you can go on to study yoga and incorporate these poses as part of your practice. If you're in a hurry, even one or two postures will lift your spirits and energy instantly. Focus on your inner body as you do these postures and continuously perform the Basic Eastern Breath.

### *The Mountain Pose*

This basic posture tones and energizes the entire body and helps you feel grounded. If you do not have that sense of rootedness, you lack the strong sense of self that allows you to "let go" to your deepest sexual feelings.

1. Stand with bare feet (if possible) hip-width apart. Focus your awareness on the sensation of being planted on the floor.
2. Lift and spread your toes, then try to bring them back to the floor one at a time, starting with the small toe and moving to the big toe. This will give you a wider foundation.
3. Starting with your ankles, and focusing on your spine, lengthen your body from the feet up, all the while maintaining that strong connection to the floor through your feet. Reach up from your ankles to your knees; from knees to hip sockets; from hips to waist; waist to shoulders. Drop your shoulders as you lengthen your neck, tilt your chin slightly in, and stretch the top of your head toward the ceiling.
4. Relax your shoulders, letting them "melt" downward away from your ears. Allow your arms to hang loosely, fingers relaxed

and soft. Like a mountain, you are rooted in the earth and reaching for the sky.

5. Add an "energetic lift" of the perineum and pelvic floor by gently contracting your "love" muscles.

### *Standing Forward Bend*

This posture helps shed stiffness, rigidity, and tension by gently stretching the entire back of the body, thus making you more limber so that you can fully articulate all the movements of sexual intercourse.

1. Assume the mountain pose stance.
2. Bend your elbows and place your hands on the crease between your thighs and hips.
3. Bending slowly and steadily from the hip sockets while keeping a straight back, lower your torso. At the same time, slide your hands down the front of your legs. Bend as far forward as you can while maintaining a straight back.
4. Hold the posture and keep performing the Basic Eastern Breath.
5. Now, allow your back to relax and let your head and neck dangle freely. Make sure that your neck, shoulders, and arms are relaxed.
6. Hold the pose, remembering to breathe, as long as you are comfortable. This is a good time to release sighs or any other tension-relieving sound.
7. When you are ready, come out of the pose by bringing your torso back up slowly, back rounded, hands on your hip sockets, until you are back in the mountain pose.

### *Seated Forward Bend*

This is an alternative posture you can do at your desk or anywhere. Because your head goes lower than your heart, it receives an increased blood supply, energizing you mentally as well as physically and giving you the vitality you need for great sex.

1. Sit in a chair about halfway forward on the seat, feet on the floor, knees about shoulder-width apart.

2. Inhale, then exhale as you allow your torso to drop forward slowly between your knees, and place both hands—one at a time—on the floor between your feet.

3. Hang limply, neck and shoulders relaxed and completely free of support.

4. Use the Basic Eastern Breath to inhale energy into any area of your body that feels tight. Exhale that stress out. Stay in the posture as long as you are comfortable.

5. Come up slowly, returning one hand to a thigh for support. Sit for a moment or two with your eyes closed, doing the Basic Eastern Breath and moving your awareness through your body to sense which parts have relaxed and which parts are still tense. Breathe into those tense areas and relax them on your exhalations.

### *Shoulder and Neck Yoga Stretches*

These stress-relieving stretches can be done anywhere, sitting or standing, and they are a wonderful way to end the day and prepare for a relaxed evening.

1. Remember not to slump. Keep your spine long, straightening and lengthening from the base.

2. Lift your shoulders and roll them in 360 degree circles to the front, up toward your ears, then back, and down. Keep breathing, sending each inhalation into a tense spot and feeling it let go as you exhale.

3. Repeat the circle several times, then do several rolls in the opposite direction.

4. Keep doing this until your shoulders feel soft and relaxed.

5. Now, stretch your neck by slowly dropping your chin toward your chest. Let your head hang free as you breathe tension out of the tight spots.

6. Slowly bring your head back to center then drop it gradually to the right side, so that your right ear is leaning over your right shoulder. Keep breathing as each exhalation gently increases the stretch. Repeat on the opposite side.

### *The Butterfly*

All of the above yoga poses will help stretch, relax, and energize your inner and outer body. The Butterfly has a more direct benefit on your sex life because it opens and softens the hip joints and stretches and tones the inner thighs—all of which is excellent preparation for sexual activity.

1. Sit on the floor and bend your knees. Bring the soles of your feet together, allowing your knees to splay open to either side of the body.
2. Take hold of your feet and draw them as close to you as possible, keeping your spine tall and shoulders relaxed.
3. Hold this pose and practice the Basic Eastern Breath, sending energy to your inner thighs and pelvic joints and letting the stretch gently increase with each long, even exhalation. If you feel any discomfort, sigh as you exhale to help release that discomfort.
4. Hold this pose as long as possible, filling your pelvic bowl with purifying air and energy and exhaling your inner thighs and hip joints further into the stretch.

### *Relaxation Pose*

Lie on your back on the floor, your feet about two feet apart, arms slightly away from your sides. If you feel any discomfort in your lower back, bend the knees and bring them together. Or roll up a pillow and place it under the knees so that the lower back relaxes into the floor and your abdomen softens.

Close your eyes and begin the Basic Eastern Breath. Turn your attention to the breath and follow its rhythms. Don't try to change anything; simply observe it. Is it slowing down? Is it becoming more shallow? Are the exhalations longer than the inhalations?

If you drop off to sleep for a while, that's okay. You can even practice this exercise in bed at night to send you off to dreamland.

Whether you fall asleep or not, you will come out of this pose feeling refreshed and energized. For those of you who find a daytime nap disorienting, the relaxation pose is a great substitute, especially when you have little time.

## TANTRIC YOGA EXERCISES

Tantric yoga views physical love as an expression of the spiritual union between male and female. Since yoga in general is about the union of opposites—yin and yang, body and mind, and so on—tantric yoga aims to reconcile the male and female principles both within you and between you and your partner. What better way to do this than through the extreme intimacy of sexual intercourse? A tantric yoga sex experience leaves you feeling deeply connected with your inner self, with your partner, and with the entire universe. The orgasms you have when practicing tantric yoga do not stop at mere genital release, and the focus of the sexual experience is not confined to the sex organs. Your entire body and mind becomes an erotic zone.

The following special exercises stimulate, strengthen, and harmonize your body, preparing it for the bliss of a tantric union.

### *Tantric Pelvis Swings*

Many Western bodywork therapies aiming to liberate the sexual energy trapped in chronic muscular tensions were inspired by the following exercise.

#### VARIATION ONE: ON ALL FOURS

1. Place your knees and palms on the floor, fingers facing forward and spread apart, thighs and arms at right angles to the floor. Your neck should extend straight from your spine, neither tipping up nor hanging down.
2. As you inhale deeply and slowly into your belly, tip your head and buttocks up, arching your back. Your belly should expand as it fills with air, and your pelvic girdle is relaxed and open.
3. Exhale slowly, at the same time tightening your buttocks and tipping your pelvis forward and under. Your back should be rounded. Feel your pelvic muscles contract and tighten.
4. Repeat this action: rhythmically inhaling, swaying your back and opening your pelvis; then exhaling as you tighten your pelvic and buttocks muscles.

With your partner: Your partner can serve as guide, touching your buttocks and stomach to guide the direction of the swings, and making sure that you are not moving any other body part, especially the thighs and middle. Your guide can also help you synchronize the inhalations and exhalations with the pelvic swings.

### Variation Two: Standing

1. Stand with legs about hip-width apart. Feel your feet planted on the floor, body weight evenly distributed between the heels and balls of your feet.
2. Lift your toes, spread them apart, then let them float down to the floor. Feel how the bottoms of your feet, including the toes, are supporting your weight.
3. Let your knees be loose and slightly flexed. Rock slightly back and forth between the front of your feet and the heels. Settle into a strong, grounded stance.
4. As you inhale air into your belly, let your pelvis swing easily backward from the "hinge" of the hips. Do not move your waist or legs, just the pelvis.
5. As you exhale, tighten the abdominals to expel the air slowly and steadily, at the same time contracting the buttocks and pushing the pelvis into a forward tilt.
6. Use your arms to help you. Allow them to dangle loosely at your sides, swinging backward with the pelvis as you inhale, then swinging forward with the pelvis as you exhale.
7. If you feel tight and "locked," that is, if your pelvis is unable to make these movements easily or without the aid of your legs or waist, keep practicing, observing your movements and correcting them in front of a mirror. Do this exercise regularly and you will loosen up.

Practice this exercise every day for five to ten minutes.

When you are able to synchronize your breathing with the pelvic rocking and arm swings, bring in your PC muscle.

As you inhale, allow your genitals to "open" and fully relax, imagining that they are filling with life-giving energy. As you exhale, contract or "lock" the PC muscle and anus to prevent the energy you have gathered from leaking out.

With your partner: Your partner can help by gently touching your hips, directing the movement of your pelvis and making sure it moves independently, without the help of any other body parts.

He or she can also guide synchronizing your breathing and pelvic locks with your hip swings.

## TAO EXERCISES

Until quite recently, many Taoist exercises and techniques were practiced only by holy men and nobility and were kept secret from the rest of the world. Although Taoist exercises have not achieved the popularity of yoga here in the West, they share many features.

Both yoga and the Tao are about the art of self healing and cultivating life-force energy, and some Taoist practices are even more effective at cultivating sexual energy than those offered by yoga. Special Taoist postures give the dedicated practitioner an astounding degree of control over his/her body, especially the ability to build and transform his/her sexual energy in ways few have ever imagined possible.

One reason Taoists cultivate sexual energy is because all the body's energy currents (also known as acupuncture meridians) pass through the pelvic area. If the pelvic area is blocked or weak, valuable life energy is lost, and all your organs and glands—even your brain—suffer.

Most of us only experience an abundance of sexual and life-force energy in our youth. We do not know how to preserve and channel this energy, let alone restore and multiply it.

Poor diet, alcohol, drugs, smoking, and excessive sex that offers only fleeting satisfaction gradually wear us out, until we either no longer desire sex or are unable to perform. We become listless, chronically tired, and even depressed.

This loss of sexual vitality and health usually takes time, so it is most often seen in middle and old age, when the pelvic and rectal muscles have weakened, sagged, and loosened, allowing vital chi energy to drain out of the body and making the older person feeble, prone to disease and dysfunction, and even senile.

However, many relatively young people suffer from loss of vital life-force energy. This makes Taoist exercises among the best remedies for the all-too-common modern-day symptoms of chronic fatigue, lack of sexual desire, impotence, infertility, lower abdominal inflammatory conditions, PMS, menstrual disorders, and other debilitating conditions, as well as for depression and other negative emotional states.

Taoist exercises strengthen and revitalize the sex organs and glands by literally increasing and concentrating their energy. The sexual energy that has been gathered is pumped from the ovaries or testicles down to the perineum, then up the spine—healing the nerves—all the way up to the brain. It is then sent down the front of the body—healing other organs and glands in its path. Finally, it travels to the navel area, where it is stored. This energy "pumping" is accomplished through a combination of breath control, visualization, and flexing of the perineum or "chi" muscles, which include the PC muscle, the root of the penis or the vaginal walls, and the anal sphincter.

## TAOIST EXERCISES AND ORGASMS

These healing exercises also allow you to orgasm either one of two ways. You can discharge through the normal, "outward" genital release, which feels wonderful, in part because it sheds tension and stress. But that release can also be accompanied by a sensation of energy depletion. An "inward" Taoist orgasm retains that aroused sexual energy in your body instead of discharging it, giving you what some people call a "valley orgasm," in which the orgasmic energy is felt in every cell of your body, at the same time that it nourishes and energizes all your organs and glands, and enhances your youthful vitality and health.

Practicing Taoist exercises and lovemaking techniques does not mean you have to give up conventional "outward" orgasms. In fact, these exercises and lovemaking techniques will work wonders on your sexual desire, performance, and "regular" orgasms, and intensify the pleasures of lovemaking overall. But you will have a degree of control over your sexuality that you never imagined possible.

If you are a woman who does not normally have orgasms, these exercises will dramatically increase your ability to orgasm. If you normally have orgasms, they will become much more intense. And while most men ejaculate with each sexual encounter, this does not mean they are enjoying the profoundly exciting and satisfying orgasms that Taoist exercises will give them.

Unless otherwise instructed, use the Basic Eastern Breath while performing all Taoist exercises.

### *Fire Belly*

This breathing exercise helps you build sexual energy by stoking the "fire" or energy contained in the area from about one inch above the pubic bone to about an inch and a half below the navel—the power center for all our body functions and activities. Practice this breath regularly and you will not only have more energy, you will become more sexually aroused in a shorter time. The Fire Belly should be performed nude.

1. Either stand feet apart and knees slightly flexed, or sit on the edge of a chair, back straight (men's genitals should be hanging free).
2. Rub the palms of your hands together briskly, until they are hot.
3. Make gentle circular motions on your lower abdomen with your left hand, covering the area from just below the navel to just above the pubic bone. Do this clockwise several times.
4. Rub your palms together to heat them up again.
5. Use your right hand to massage the same area several times in a counterclockwise motion.
6. Inhale and exhale evenly, making sure to breathe deep into your pelvis.

Make as many circles as you wish, making sure that you rub an equal number of times in each direction.

### *Hip and Sacrum Loosener*

If your hip bones and the sacrum (the fused group of vertebrae that forms the base of the spine) are not exercised properly, they will fuse together over time, inhibiting the mobility you need to become fully aroused. Practice this exercise regularly, and you will gradually separate the hips from the sacrum and restore the level of pelvic flexibility that is essential for building and discharging powerful sexual passion.

1. Stand with your feet planted firmly on the floor, hip-width apart, knees slightly flexed.
2. Place your hands on your hips to hold them still as you focus on moving your sacrum only, forward and back.

Or you can ask your partner to place one hand on your sacrum and the other on your hip, making sure that only your sacrum moves.

### *The Kidney Stimulator*

The Kidney Stimulator strengthens the kidneys and adrenals and the glandular system, thereby increasing sexual desire and even relieving lower back pain. The exercise is also prescribed by Taoist healers to counter impotence and premature ejaculation and keep the skin smooth and beautiful.

1. Sit or lie down comfortably. Rub the palms together briskly until they are very warm.
2. Place your palms on the small of your back as you tilt your upper body slightly forward. Feel and visualize the energy flowing from your hands into your kidneys and adrenals.
3. Massage the small of your back by rubbing up and down and then in a circular motion.
4. Now, make a loose fist and softly pummel the small of your back for a few seconds.
5. Repeat the rubbing and pummeling three times.

### *The Deer*

This basic but powerfully effective Taoist exercise for men and women increases and balances endocrine gland secretions and boosts energy levels. When your sex glands function at optimum levels, sexual desire is high, and your entire being feels energized, toned, and rejuvenated.

The Deer is also based on the principle that the foundation of good health and lifelong sexual vitality are strong, toned anal muscles. When you exercise your anal sphincter, the male prostate gland, which lies behind the anal muscles, automatically receives toning benefits, thereby helping to protect the prostate from enlargement, inflammation, and other dysfunctions that plague so many men over fifty. These exercises also tone women's vaginal muscles, benefiting the uterus and ovaries and helping to prevent many common maladies of the female sex organs and glands, including the symptoms of menopause. The Deer also helps prevent and cure hemorrhoids in both sexes.

### Male Deer Exercise

The Male Deer exercise can help overcome impotence and premature ejaculation and is even said to enlarge the head of the penis!

Do this exercise in the nude, preferably after bathing:

1. Sit forward on a chair so that your testicles hang free.
2. Rub the palms of your hands together briskly until you feel a build-up of heat.
3. Cupping your testicles gently with your right hand, close your eyes and feel heat enter and energize your testicles.
4. Keeping your right hand cupped over your scrotum, place your left palm gently over the pubic area, beginning one inch below your navel. Circle that area clockwise, several times. Repeat in a counterclockwise direction an equal number of times. Do this as many times as comfortable, rubbing your palms together whenever they cool down.

If this abdominal massage is too difficult to perform in combination with the following steps, wait to introduce the abdominal massage until you are more practiced and comfortable.

5. Squeeze the PC and anal muscles together. Hold the contraction as long as you're comfortable, then relax those muscles. Repeat, making sure to rest between contractions.

After several weeks of daily practice, you will be able to contract the PC and anal muscles for a longer period.

This contraction of the area from ureter to anus is called a "lock" or "energetic lift." It is key to many Taoist exercises because it closes off the trunk of the body, allowing you to retain the sexual energy you've built up, instead of letting it "leak out."

Without control over the PC and anal muscles, Taoists believe it is impossible to strengthen and energize your sex glands and organs, as well as the rest of your body.

Once you have control over these muscles, you can use the "lock" in combination with the massage part of this exercise.

Practice the Deer in the morning and evening. If you get an erection, place the thumb of your right hand, which is cupping the testicles, at the base of your penis, next to the pubic bone. Press down sharply, at the same time massaging the pubic bone with your left hand. This stops blood from flowing into and erecting your penis. You don't want to discharge the sexual energy you've cultivated through an orgasm. Instead, you are trying to gather and conserve energy in order to stimulate and tone the sex organs and glands.

As you become more proficient, you will learn how to move the sexual energy you've cultivated up your spine, transforming it into a revitalizing force for your entire body.

### Female Deer Exercise

Women should also practice the Deer after bathing and in the nude. Regular practice of this exercise helps prevent and even cure a host of sex organ and gland-related problems. It is also a wonderful way to maintain youthful sexual energy and beauty.

Women add a "vaginal lock" to their PC/anal contraction.

1. Sit on the floor, a couch, or bed and draw the heel of one foot up to your groin so that it presses against the opening of your vagina and your clitoris. It your heel won't reach, place a hard round object, such as a child's ball (covered by a clean cloth), against the area, until you feel a gentle, pleasurably stimulating pressure.
2. Rub your palms together briskly to build up heat, then cover your breasts with your hands and feel the heat penetrate every cell.
3. Now, rub your breasts gently but firmly in an outward, circular motion. Move the right hand in a clockwise direction; the left in a counterclockwise direction. Taoists recommend doing this for a minimum of 36 circles and a maximum of 306 circles, but

you can circle as many times as you wish, making sure to circle in each direction an equal number of times. This outward massage clears congestion, preventing and even curing lumps.

4. Rub your hands together briskly again. Reverse direction, rubbing your breasts in an inward, circular motion (right, counterclockwise; left, clockwise) to stimulate them. This direction increases their size and firmness.

Together with the pressure on your clitoris and groin, the breast massage builds a warm sexual excitement that stimulates hormone production.

5. Now, tighten your anal and vaginal muscles and hold the lock as long as comfortable. Relax, then repeat.

After weeks of regular practice, you should be able to hold the contraction for a longer period. When you gain more control, you will be able to do the locks while rubbing your breasts.

Eventually you will learn how to move the energy you've gathered up your spine to your brain and then down the front of your body, healing and revitalizing every organ and gland in its path.

### *Egg Exercises*

These exercises, until recently a secret known only to the courtesans and rulers of imperial China, are practiced with a stone or wooden egg. They, and the remaining exercises in this chapter, are adapted from *Healing Love Through the Tao: Cultivating Female Sexual Energy* by Mantak Chia and Maneewan Chia. (See Resource Guide, page 259.) The "eggs" used for these exercises can be ordered from a mail order company (also listed in the Resource Guide, page 262). Though they may sound outlandish at first, the strength, agility, and control—not to mention lifelong sexual health and youthful beauty—that is gained from their regular practice is more than worth the effort. Your increased tone and sensitivity will keep your hormones balanced, your libido healthy, and your orgasms satisfying.

Most women use an egg about one inch in diameter, but the smaller the egg, the more your muscles have to work.

Make sure that your vagina and the egg are clean. A stone egg will attract less bacteria than one made of wood, but it is essential that the egg is immersed for five minutes in boiling water before using it for the first time, then wash it with a nonallergenic, non-irritating soap before and after each subsequent use.

Do not use the egg unless the vagina is lubricated. This means that you will have to arouse yourself before exercising. You can use the Deer for this purpose. If needed, use a water-based lubricant. Always insert the larger or wider end of the egg first.

Your mind power is key in the egg exercises, as many of the muscles involved are involuntary ones over which you will acquire unprecedented control.

Throughout the exercises, always keep the vaginal opening contracted. To remove the egg, squeeze as if you were having a bowel movement and the egg will come out. (If it gets stuck, just lie down and squeeze it out.)

Place a cushion or towel under your feet, because the egg can drop out and break.

1. Insert the egg, then take the stance used for all the egg exercises: feet hip-width apart, ankles and knees slightly bent, spine straight.
2. Raise your arms until they extend straight in front of you, palms up. Clench your fists.
3. Inhale as you contract the first third (outer) of your vagina. Concentrate on isolating the muscles that close and tighten the vaginal opening and on keeping the egg in the vaginal canal.
4. Inhale again and concentrate on tightening the middle section of the vagina as well.
5. Inhale and tighten the upper third section, so that you are now contracting the entire vaginal canal.
6. Inhale and squeeze the egg, moving it to the middle section of your vagina. Inhale and squeeze, increasing the pressure. Inhale again and squeeze even harder.
7. Maintaining your grip, try to move the egg up and down the vagina. Start with a slow, even motion. If you pick up speed, do not lose the steady rhythm. When you are tired, rest.
8. Feel energy building in the vagina during resting periods.

After you have mastered moving the egg up and down, go on to the next step:

9. Keeping the egg in the middle section, move it to the left and right.

10. Bring the egg to the upper section of your vagina and then move it left and right.

11. When you have mastered these two previous steps, move the egg down to the first or outer section of the vagina, then move it left and right.

12. After you have mastered all of the previous steps, move the egg left and right and up and down. Master this step before continuing to the next movements.

13. Tilt the egg up and down, moving between the top and the outer part of your vagina. Practice until you have mastered this action.

14. Now, combine all the movements, moving the egg left and right, tilting it up and down, moving it up to touch the cervix, and then down to the external vaginal orifice. Rest and feel the energy that you've built up.

Practice your egg exercises for a few minutes at a time, two to three times a week, gradually increasing the length of time you keep the egg moving inside you.

After you can make all these movements fairly easily, practice the same movements without the egg.

You can also try to suck up the egg, that is, pull it into your vagina off a chair seat with Hooverlike force!

### *Two Egg Exercises*

Once you have accomplished the single egg exercises, you can try inserting two eggs at the same time. Try moving them in opposite directions—one up, one down—as well as banging them together to set off a vibration that stimulates your sex organs and glands.

### *Vaginal Weight-lifting*

Yes, the idea is mind-boggling, but, once again, the benefits to your sexual health and pleasure are immeasurable.

You need a wooden egg for this exercise, about one inch in diameter, with a hole drilled all the way through so you can thread a string that you then attach to a weight. You will also need a half pound weight with a hole in the center through which you thread the string. Or you can place the weight in a small, drawstring bag.

You do not move the egg up and down in these exercises. Instead, hold the egg in place by contracting the first two thirds of the vaginal canal and pulling the egg upward. Do not release your grip.

Perform this exercise two to three times a week, gradually increasing the weight in half-pound increments, never going beyond ten pounds. Do it while standing in the basic egg exercise posture, with the seat of a chair positioned under your genitals.

1. Make sure you are lubricated, then insert the egg, large end first, while you hold the string and weight in your other hand. Use a sucking force to position the egg securely.
2. Place the weight on the seat of the chair.
3. Grip the egg using the muscles of the vagina. Let go of the string and weight, keeping your hand just underneath, in case it falls out.
4. Inhale and contract the vagina even more tightly. At the same time, use the power of your mind to contract your uterus.
5. Inhale and visualize pulling the weight up by the cervix. Holding your breath, contract even harder.
6. When you feel your grip is secure, begin gently rocking your pelvis so that the weight swings forward and back. Do this thirty to sixty times.
7. When you've built up a lot of energy, inhale all the way down to your ovaries, gathering their energy and bringing it into the uterus and then to the clitoris. Hold it there.
8. Inhale and use your mind to pull all the energy you have gathered down to the perineum, then up the spine and into your brain, all the while holding the egg inside the deepest portion of your vagina. Hold your breath and continue sending energy up your spine with each inhalation.
9. Place your tongue against the roof of your mouth. Exhale, and allow the energy you've gathered to flow down the front of your body until it reaches your navel.
10. Rest the weight on the chair and push the egg out, catching it in your hand.

11. Gently massage your pelvic region, including your sacrum, to help your body absorb the energy.

12. Since a wooden egg attracts more bacteria, be sure to wash it thoroughly after each use and before using it again.

### *Taoist Sex Organ Energizer*

This exercise is designed to tone and stimulate the sex organs and glands by pressing the vital life-force energy in your upper body down into your pelvis. Once you have mastered this exercise and the Taoist Energy Transformation exercise that follows, you will become more easily and rapidly aroused, and you will enjoy far more intensely pleasurable orgasms.

1. Sit in a comfortable cross-legged position or on a straight-back chair.

2. Inhale deeply through your nose, sending energy into your throat, as you touch your tongue to the roof of your mouth.

3. Swallow the air, then drive it down to your solar plexus (between your heart and navel), then on to your ovaries, uterus, and vagina/penis and scrotum, where you gather and compress this energy. Do this by contracting your abs in a downward, wave-like movement.

   Visualize this air as a ball of energy you are rolling down your abdomen and packing into your sex organs and glands.

4. As you push down and pack life-force energy into your sex organs and glands, activate your PC/anal lock to keep the energy from escaping. Your sex organs should feel as if they're being filled and heated up.

5. Now, exhale and relax, making sure to swallow any saliva that has accumulated in your mouth.

6. Work up to compressions that last thirty, then forty, then sixty seconds long.

This exercise brings immediate results. If you feel lethargic, ill, or tired, do several Taoist Sex Organ Energizers, and you'll be restored in no time.

### *Taoist Energy Transformation*

This powerful exercise brings together three elements: the breath, the PC/anal or "love" muscles, and the power of your mind. It builds and gathers the concentrated life-force energy stored in the ovaries/testicles, then draws it up the body, where it delivers vitality and healing. It can take some time to master, but once you have, all you will have to do is direct your sexual energy with your mind, and your body will respond immediately. Take all the time you need to learn this exercise—several days to weeks to months—and don't skip any steps. It will do wonders to increase your sexual voltage and transform that energy into a powerful healing force. It is best done in the nude.

1. Sit cross-legged and rub the palms of your hands together vigorously until they feel hot.
2. Practice the Deer.
3. Caress your body, feeling the heat and energy from your palms penetrate your skin and warm the inside of your body.
4. Bring your arousal level to the point of orgasm.
5. When you are near to or in the midst of orgasm, inhale deeply through your nose. At the same time, contract all your muscles—clenching the fists, clawing the feet down, clenching the jaw, tightening the back of the neck, and pressing the tongue firmly against the roof of the mouth.

   Activate the lock.
6. Do this several times, always maintaining your anal/PC muscle locks to secure the sexual energy.
7. Whenever you're out of breath, exhale and feel the energy building in your sex organs.
8. Inhale and hold your breath at the same time that you begin to rhythmically squeeze and relax the anal and PC muscles in a pumping action.
9. As you pump, see your sexual energy as a golden light concentrating in your genitals. After each pump, exhale and relax.
10. Inhale once more as you activate your locks and pull the golden light from the sex organs down to the perineum (the midpoint between the urinary opening and the anus).
11. Inhale once again and pull the golden light to the base of the spine. On your next inhalation, move it to the middle of the back, then to the neck, until, finally, it reaches the top of your head. If, at any point in this process, you feel the energy level lowering, stop to rebuild your arousal by pumping.

12. Circle the energy in your brain several times, first clockwise, then counterclockwise.

13. Touch the front of the tongue to the roof of the mouth. Stop pumping and feel the energy you have generated flow down the front of your body from the crown of the head, past the nose, mouth, throat, heart, chest, and then into the navel area, thereby making a complete circuit of energy.

### *Genital Sunbathing*

This practice draws the powerful life-force energy of the sun into the body. It is especially energizing for women because their genital organs are mostly internal. If you have a sunny area with privacy, practice genital sunbathing for no more than twenty to thirty minutes at a time, as damage to the ozone layer has made excessive sunbathing harmful to your health. The safest times are between seven and eleven in the morning and three and six in the afternoon, when the sun's rays are less powerful.

A woman can lie on her back, drawing the soles of the feet together, so that the knees are splayed open, exposing the genitals to the sun. The hands are tucked under the lower back, palms down, thumbs touching. This position circulates the energy absorbed from the sun throughout the body.

A man absorbs the sun's energy through the head of his penis. The best position is lying on the back, lower body facing the sun. Holding the stem of the penis with one hand, he stimulates himself to erection, then allows the sun's power to enter through the head of the penis. While in this position, he can also pull his testicles up to expose them to the sun's healing rays.

### *Taoist Sitz Baths*

#### COLD-WATER SITZ BATH

Immersing the lower body in cold water increases blood flow to the sex organs and glands, stimulating the prostate and sperm production in men and hormone production in women. Squat or sit in a tub of cold water, so that your genitals, anus, and the bottom of your spine are immersed, for ten to twenty minutes.

Start off with cool water and gradually get yourself accustomed to colder temperatures.

### Alternating Hot and Cold Sitz Baths

Use two plastic sitz baths or washtubs, filling one with hot water and the other with cold. Immerse your lower body first in hot then in cold water in order to increase blood circulation, tone the body, increase resistance to disease, and stimulate hormone production. You can lower yourself in gradually, but stay in each bath for a minimum of three minutes before switching. Alternate between the hot and cold baths at least six times and make sure your entire lower trunk is immersed. If you don't have time for these baths, you can shower in hot water and rinse off in cold.

### Air Baths

Exposing the bare skin to fresh air builds the body's resistance to disease and improves blood circulation. It also keeps the male genitals cooler than the rest of the body, thus protecting the sperm. This is also a wonderfully sensuous and liberating experience. Make sure you have privacy and that the weather is warm enough. You can also take an air bath in your home by sitting near wide-open windows.

## Acupressure and Acupuncture

Acupuncture and acupressure are more popular today than ever before, and many conventional medical doctors are incorporating these ancient healing systems into their practices. Acupuncture schools are opening up all over the country and licensing boards have been set up in most states to regulate practitioners and protect clients.

Both acupuncture and acupressure are based on a detailed energy map of the human body that locates the precise channels (known as meridians) through which life-force energy travels and connects every body part. All disease, weakness, and dysfunction, including those affecting sexuality, are thought to be caused by blockages of life-force energy that cause either energy stagnation or energy deficiency in various organ and gland systems.

Acupuncture and acupressure heal by locating these energy blockages and either inserting fine needles into or applying pressure over specific points to free blockages and restore proper energy flow and health.

Even if your physical problem is due to chronic tension, acupuncture or acupressure can relieve the effects of stress on your body and restore healthy blood and energy circulation.

## ACUPRESSURE

Acupressure, or the Japanese term "shiatsu," consists of finger pressure applied to specific points in order to unblock life-force energy. The result is stimulated circulation, relief from pain, and revitalization of your entire being. Since all traditional Eastern healing systems view the body as an integrated whole, virtually any blockage in the body will have an adverse effect on sexual health and impair sexual pleasure.

If your sex life is below par, whether your problem is physical or mental in origin, acupressure can help. It may be more pleasurable to have someone work on you, but you can also do it yourself any time, at your convenience, and you don't have to pay a single cent.

### *How to Apply Self-Acupressure*

Always use firm pressure to stimulate the body's natural curative abilities. It will hurt a bit—especially if you need treatment on a particular point. But this slight pain should feel "sweet," as the Japanese describe the healing sensation.

You can use your thumb, finger, palm, the side of a hand, or your knuckles to apply the pressure. Some professional acupressure practitioners even use their feet and elbows.

Use prolonged, steady pressure; three minutes per point is ideal.

### *Points for Sexual Vitality*

#### Sea of Vitality

Location: Altogether, these comprise four points located on the lower back, two and four finger-widths away from the spine on either side, at waist level.

Benefits: relieves lower back aches, fatigue, sexual-reproductive problems, impotency, and premature ejaculation.

#### Bubbling Springs

Location: On the center of the sole of the foot, at the base of the ball of the foot, between the two pads.

Benefits: Relieves hot flashes and impotency.

#### Bigger Stream

Location: Midway between the inside ankle bone and the Achilles tendon, on the back of the ankle.

Benefits: Relieves sexual tensions, semen leakage, menstrual irregularity, and fatigue.

Caution: Do not use this point after the third month of pregnancy.

#### Three Mile Point

Location: Four finger-widths below the kneecap, one finger-width on the outside of the shinbone. If you are on the correct spot, a muscle should flex under your finger as you move your foot up and down.

Benefits: Strengthens entire body, especially the muscles, and aids the sexual-reproductive systems. It normally takes months of daily practice to relieve impotency.

#### Gate Origin

Location: Four finger-widths directly below the belly button.

Benefits: Relieves impotency, reproductive problems, irregular vaginal discharge, irregular menstrual periods, and urinary incontinence.

### ACUPUNCTURE

Simply put, acupuncture is a stronger version of acupressure. A certified acupuncturist can determine which points should be penetrated by needles in order to release blocked energy and restore balanced energy flow and vitality.

The needles may look lethal to a novice, but acupuncture is painless and promotes a pleasant sensation of well-being. The needles are usually left in for fifteen to twenty minutes and are said by practitioners to also attract healing energy from the universe into the body.

## WESTERN BODYWORK AND THERAPEUTIC TOUCH THERAPIES

All of the following Western bodywork systems owe a good deal to traditional Asian disciplines in that they spring from the underlying premise that human beings are holistic entities whose vitality depends on the free flow of life-force energy. Also fundamental to these bodywork systems is the belief that physical health, emotional stability, spiritual awareness, and sexuality are interconnected in profound and basic ways.

### ROLFING

Ida Rolf is the founder of all the Western bodywork systems that loosen the body's muscular structure in order to restore balance, sensation, and free movement. Rolfing goes deep into the muscle to loosen the fascia tissue that covers muscles and, if rigid, restricts movement and sensation.

Rolfing, and all the Western bodywork techniques that developed from it, links rigidities in the body's musculature with a person's inability to tolerate deep emotion and physical pleasure, particularly such powerful and primal emotions as fear, passion, and rage, as well as sexual desire and pleasure.

The body literally stores repressed emotion by contracting the very same muscles it would use to express that emotion. Over time, repeated and chronic contractions cause fascia and muscle tissue to become rigid and wrinkled. It becomes virtually impossible to fully breathe and experience bodily sensations, especially the thrill of sexual excitement flooding your body. Numbed by these chronic muscular contractions, you also are unable to release yourself to the overwhelming experience of a powerful orgasm, which is a series of rhythmic contractions and relaxations experienced throughout your body. This is especially true if your pelvic and abdominal muscles are rigid, in effect "armored" against deep feeling and sensation.

The aim of Rolfing is to free your body from the prison of these rigid muscles so that it becomes more balanced, efficient, and relaxed, and your full capacity for sexual function and pleasure is restored.

The Rolfer uses his or her fingers, fists, and elbows to probe beyond the body's soft tissue and stretch out the stiffened muscles and fascia. Muscles and soft tissue are separated and freed. Your body becomes aligned and more flexible. While you may not resolve emotional issues concerning sexual repression and trauma, they will no longer be stored in your body. You become more open, better able to tolerate and express deep emotion, including profound sexual pleasure and the powerful sensations of orgasm.

Basic treatment takes ten sessions. Rolfing can be quite painful when the practitioner is working on especially rigid areas. But the pain is "sweet," because you are also experiencing a profound physical—and sometimes emotional—release.

## FELDENKRAIS

Developed by an Israeli engineer/physicist, Feldenkrais emphasizes movement re-education. The practitioner coaches the client so that his or her body awareness and sense of balance is heightened. The basic theory is that movement and the nervous system are inextricably linked, so the brain is "retrained" to correct the body's inefficient and harmful habits.

A major harmful habit is to hold the abdominal and pelvic muscles in chronic contractions, in order to conform to our cultural ideal of a flat tummy. However, that spastic contraction also creates a numbing effect, cutting us off from deep sexual feelings.

Treatment consists of the practitioner gently rocking the client's arms, legs, hinges, and joints over and over, for six to ten sessions, thereby retraining the client to use his/her body in a more balanced, efficient manner.

## ALEXANDER TECHNIQUE

The Alexander Technique was developed by a Shakespearian actor around the turn of the last century. The Alexander Technique is similar to Feldenkrais in that the brain and body are "retrained" to use the body more efficiently, thereby allowing it to soften any harmful muscular contractions on its own. The Alexander Technique practitioner is more of a coach and the client is more active—walking, sitting, standing, etc.—as the practitioner helps him or her focus awareness on all body movements and posture patterns involved. The client gradually learns which produce tension and fatigue and replaces them with newer, more productive ways to move and hold his or her body. Sessions are often ongoing, with some people having two sessions per week.

# 5

# THE BODY-MIND-SEX CONNECTION

The last chapter described traditional Eastern exercises and modern Western exercises that strengthen, tone, and make your body more flexible—even soften any muscular "armor" that could block your sexual pleasure. This chapter extends the holistic approach to improving your sex life to include your mind—the most powerful sex organ of all.

As we explore the body-mind-sex connection, you will learn more about how suppressed emotions can stand in the way of your full sexual expression and happiness. You will discover how negative and self-limiting thoughts about your sexuality can numb your capacity for sensuous pleasure, creating a devastating ripple effect that prevents you from tolerating the build-up of a powerful sexual charge and its explosive orgasmic release.

This chapter will also teach you how to use relaxation and visualization techniques to counter any self-limiting thoughts you might have regarding your sexuality. And if you think you lack enough imagination to do these visualizations, you can practice exercises described here that will put you more in touch with this natural facility.

## Reichian and Bioenergetic Theory and Practice

As you learned in the last chapter, the same muscles used to express an emotion are the very ones you contract to shut that emotion down. These buried feelings can include any early trauma that induced terror, grief, or sexual shame. Those traumas and emotions don't just go away. They are simply held in check by the viselike grip of your rigid muscles. Imagine how much vitality is lost after years, even decades, of expending your energy in the ongoing struggle to keep those feelings suppressed.

Even if repressed emotions are not directly related to your sexuality, the near-permanent muscular contractions they create inhibit your capacity for full sexual pleasure and release. The seat of deep emotion—fear, rage, sorrow—is the pelvic area. So, whenever we deny any deep feeling, we automatically restrict our ability to feel the profound pleasures of sexual sensation. In other words, your unexpressed, long-forgotten emotions can hold your body—and your sexuality!—hostage.

When those rigid muscles are released through special breathing and physical exercises, their accompanying emotions are also freed and your true sexual nature is liberated.

Reichian therapy and its offshoots—bioenergetics and other body-mind therapies—include exercises designed to liberate you from your muscular defense system or "armor." When muscular contractions (especially those constricting pelvic and abdominal movement) are released, you are able to tolerate a far deeper level of sexual excitement and orgasmic intensity. In these exercises, as in the traditional Eastern techniques that inspired Reich and other Westerners, the first step toward fulfilling your sexual potential is the breath.

In his seminal book, *The Function of the Orgasm*, Wilhelm Reich states:

> The most important means of bringing about the orgasm reflex is a *breathing technique* [italics added]. . . . There is no neurotic individual who is capable of exhaling in one breath, deeply and evenly. The patients have developed all conceivable practices which prevent *deep expiration* [italics added]. They exhale "jerkily," or, as soon as the air is let out, they quickly bring their chest back into inspiratory position. . . .
>
> The sensation of this inhibition is localized in the upper abdomen or in the middle of the abdomen. With deep expi-

ration, there appear in the abdomen vivid sensations of pleasure or anxiety. . . . *Deep expiration brings about spontaneously the attitude of (sexual) surrender* [italics added].

Reich also talks about "the mobilization of the dead pelvis" as the primary way to release suppressed emotions and increase capacity for full sexual pleasure and release.

The armored pelvis is the main reason why most men and women today cannot tolerate strong sexual passion. Unable to breathe deep into their bellies or execute the smooth, natural pelvic movements of sexual union *that should be involuntary,* most American men and women cannot build a powerful sexual charge, let alone release that charge freely and utterly.

"The immobility of the pelvis gives the impression of deadness," Reich wrote. "In the majority of cases, this is subjectively felt as an 'emptiness in the pelvis' or a 'weakness of the genitals.' " He also linked "holding back in the pelvis" to chronic constipation. Because "the pelvis has lost its natural motility," Reich added, "such patients always suffer from a severe disturbance of the sexual act. The women lie motionless, or else they try to overcome the blocking of the vegetative motility by forced movements of the trunk and pelvis together. In men, the same disturbance takes the form of quick, hasty, and voluntary movements of all of the lower body. . . . The genital musculature is tense, so that the contractions which normally take place as a response to friction cannot occur."

Reich goes on to detail the positions in which these "deadened" pelvises are typically frozen, then concludes that "it is possible to deaden any genital pleasure sensation by a chronic contracture of the pelvis musculature. . . . The most important and most common of the voluntary movements [of the pelvis] is that of moving abdomen, pelvis, and thighs *in one piece* [italics added]. It is perfectly useless to have the patient do exercises with his pelvis, as many gymnastic teachers intuitively do. As long as the concealing and defensive attitudes and actions are not discovered and eliminated, the natural pelvic movement cannot develop."

Modern sex research and writing tends to focus on women's inability to orgasm or orgasm vaginally, that is, through penile-vaginal intercourse. But this pelvic "deadening" applies just as much to men. The fact that most men ejaculate does not mean they are experiencing the all-consuming ecstasy of a true orgasm. It's as if their penises were separate entities from the rest of their bodies. They "get off," but they never let go.

As noted earlier, Caribbean people prize their natural ability to "wind the waistline," that is, move the pelvis and torso with supple freedom. Unfortunately, many Americans lack the freedom of this flexibility. Our torsos tend to be immobile, rigid from the chest to the knees, even when we are well-trained in various forms of dance. Stiff and unyielding, we are unable to release our bodies to the natural pelvic undulations that mark uninhibited, passionate sex. In other words, we are not feeling all that we can feel.

In *The Betrayal of the Body,* Alexander Lowen, M.D., the founder of Reichian offshoot bioenergetic therapy, concurs with Reich when he writes, "A body is forsaken when it becomes a source of pain and humiliation instead of pleasure and pride." In contrast, "the alive body . . . is manifested by the spontaneity of its gestures and the vivacity of its expression. . . . I have repeatedly stressed how afraid people are to feel their bodies. On some level they are aware that the body is a repository of their repressed feelings, and while they would very much like to know about these repressed feelings, they are loathe to encounter them in the flesh . . . afraid of love and orgasm . . . afraid to let his body go."

Lowen describes a "well-integrated and coordinated body" as functioning "like a bow in many activities. The pitcher throwing a ball, the woodcutter swinging an ax. . . . The sexual movements are also based on this principle. Any disturbance which hinders the body from moving according to this principle will decrease the ability of the person to achieve full orgastic satisfaction."

## BIOENERGETIC EXERCISES

Lowen developed exercises to release the rigid musculature that binds deep sexual passion and prevents us from feeling fully grounded, vital, and passionate. These exercises help integrate body and mind by softening the muscular armor that developed to protect the person from emotional or physical pain—particularly in the vulnerable pelvic and abdominal areas that are the seat of sexual feelings.

Bioenergetic exercises also encourage the body to engage in the movements and postures associated with deep natural breathing, complete physical mobility, and profound sexual release.

Warning: If you feel as though recovering suppressed emotions and/or past experiences could be too overwhelming to handle alone, do this with the help of a skilled body-mind therapist. For many of you, though, emotional and physical release will come as a great relief.

### *The Bioenergetic Stool*

A "bioenergetic stool" can be made from a common kitchen stool that reaches waist-high. Cut down the legs if yours is too tall. If the seat is not padded, cover it with layers of foam and then a piece of material secured to the underside of the seat with tacks or staples.

Bending backward over the stool opens and deepens your breathing and makes your torso more stretched and flexible, thereby preparing you to tolerate and enjoy the build-up and release of powerful sexual feelings.

1. Stand with your back to the stool.
2. Bend your knees, remembering to keep your feet planted firmly on the floor, at least shoulder-width apart. Gradually and carefully lean back, so you are arched backward, your back supported by the stool with your lower spine and pelvis free.
3. Your arms should be overhead, your hands grasping a ledge—a window sill or counter, for example. This gives you added stretch and support.
4. Feel the muscles of your abdomen and back stretch and release tension. Feel your breathing automatically deepen.
5. Allow your head to hang back loosely. Jut your jaw forward and begin taking long, deep inhalations through your nose and mouth.
6. Feel these inhalations fill your entire body, especially the pelvic bowl. Your muscles will soften and release further with each long exhalation. Make these exhalations deep, heart-felt sighs. The more often you sigh and the longer and louder they are, the more years—even decades—you will shed of muscular and emotional pain, constriction, and tension.

7. Imagine your pelvis is a balloon that swells larger and softens more each time you exhale and release tension.

8. Feel your body let go and stretch; feel the tight muscles in the front of your thighs loosen and lengthen.

9. After your body becomes more relaxed, your pelvis should begin to swing back and forth spontaneously: backward as you inhale and forward as you exhale. These involuntary movements are key to releasing long-held tension. They are also the natural movements of sex and orgasm.

The more fully you inhale and exhale, the more feelings will come up to be expressed. As this continues to happen, your pelvic armor loosens more and more and vital energy begins to fill your body.

You are beginning to feel alive and complete in a way you've never felt before.

All sorts of feelings might emerge: fear, sadness, anger, sexual desire, as well as a delicious sense of connectedness, of being whole, complete, and fully present in your body. Express any feelings that emerge through sounds. If tears come, don't worry. These tears will fill you with a sweet melancholy, as you reexperience past pain for a few brief moments, then let it go. The more you give in to these feelings, the quicker they will pass from you, leaving you refreshed, energized, softened, and free to enjoy your true sexuality.

Soon, you will feel energy—a sensation similar to pins and needles—streaming up from your feet to your legs, pelvis, chest, neck, head. Keep breathing and rocking your pelvis, until this sensation of aliveness engulfs your entire body. Enjoy the marvelous feeling of your natural vitality.

10. To come up from the stool, let go of the ledge, bend your elbows, and place one hand at the back of your head. Use the other hand to push forward, so that you come out of your stretch.

Go over your stool for five to ten minutes or more every day or so, and you will soon observe that your ability to breathe fully and freely increases dramatically, along with your capacity to enjoy the sensations of your body. You will move from here to the next exercise, which counterbalances the backward stretch.

Each time you bend back over the stool, do the following forward-bending exercise to reverse the stretch.

### *Forward Bend*

1. Keeping your feet planted firmly on the ground about shoulder-width apart, turn your toes slightly inward, so that you are slightly pigeon-toed. Allow your knees to soften and flex slightly.

2. Let your trunk bend forward so that it hangs freely over your legs. Do not try to bring your trunk close to your thighs; just let your upper body hang loosely and easily. Your knees are soft and slightly flexed, toes slightly inward and supporting your entire body weight. Allow your fingers to lightly graze the ground for balance.

3. Adjust the degree of flexion in your knees so that you feel a stretch at the backs of your legs and thighs.

4. Your abdomen is loose, so your breathing should automatically deepen. Focus your awareness on the tension in your calf muscles and hamstrings and on the contact between your feet and the floor.

5. Keep breathing slowly and evenly. Eventually, you will feel a tremor in your legs. As you continue to breathe, the tremor will increase and spread upward. The tingling will feel exactly like the "pins and needles" sensation of the previous exercise. A wonderful sense of aliveness fills your pelvis, awakening your sexuality, then spreads to engulf your entire body.

If you want to speed up the streaming of energy through your body, gently and rhythmically pump your knees as you continue to inhale and exhale, deeply and rhythmically. Do not allow your knees to straighten completely, or "lock," as this will cut off the upward flow of energy.

### *Lying Down Leg Pump*

A variation of the above exercise can be done on the floor.

1. Lie on your back.

2. Inhale, then exhale as you press your lower spine into the floor, tilting the pelvis upward. Do this a few times to loosen your lower back and prevent strain.

3. Bring both legs straight up and take hold of your toes, left

hand gripping left toes and right hand gripping right toes. Keeping your knees slightly bent, extend your heels to the ceiling to stretch your calf muscles and hamstrings.

4. Breathe deeply and slowly, in and out, allowing any sounds to release on the exhalations.

5. Begin pumping your legs slightly. Inhale as you bend them slightly and exhale as you straighten them (but never completely). Keep your heels extended and stretched. Pump evenly until the "streaming," or pins and needles sensation, begins in your feet and courses up your body in waves. Keep breathing deeply, making any sounds that emerge and pumping when needed, until the sensation of life-force energy fills your entire body.

6. Release your legs and let them drift down to the floor.

7. Gently roll onto your side into a comfortable position. Rest a few moments, then roll up on your knees and bring yourself into a seated or standing position.

Note: All of the above exercises can be done with the help of a partner. You can help each other over and up from the stool, guide each other's pelvic rocking, remind each other to breathe deeply, to make sounds, and support each other in staying with the exercise, especially when an uncomfortable feeling comes up to be released.

## Guided Visualizations

Try this simple exercise. Close your eyes and make your mind an absolute blank for a few moments.

What is happening? Does your attention keep wandering to the sounds of traffic outside, the wind rustling in the trees, the list of chores you must complete today, that argument you had with your friend last week, the rumbling in your tummy that tells you it's time for lunch?

If all this interference is sullying that perfect blankness you're aiming for, don't worry. You're normal. Only seasoned meditators can observe that passing parade of mind-talk with distance and objectivity. And that takes a lot of practice.

That's one reason why we use guided visualizations instead of meditation. Instead of letting your mind wander wherever it will, guided visualizations provide a script it can follow. The script is tailored specifically to you, written with the goal of liberating you from any thoughts and belief systems that are inhibiting your sex life, so that you can go on to create a happier sexual reality for yourself.

If you can visualize in precise detail all the changes you want in your sex life—painting a vivid mental picture of your sex life just as you wish it to be—almost by magic, your sexual reality will begin conforming to that image.

## Relaxation Techniques

Before you can reap the benefits of guided visualizations, you must first learn to relax as completely as possible. You can accept and incorporate alternative beliefs much more easily when you are relaxed. You are more open for "reprogramming," for taking in suggestions on new patterns of thought and behavior regarding your sexuality that will eventually replace the negative thoughts and behaviors.

Relaxation training begins with focusing on the breath and muscle relaxation and then progresses to allowing thoughts to drift into the mind, rather than hanging onto any worrisome thoughts that are already there. In this relaxed state, you can distance yourself from negative thoughts and emotions about your sexuality and make room for the positive images of the guided visualization.

The ideal mind state for a guided visualization is one of relaxed attention: you are alert and concentrated on what is happening inside you, but, at the same time, uninvolved with what may be happening on the outside.

It is important to understand that this kind of relaxation means time alone in a quiet environment where you will not be disturbed, even by the telephone or doorbell. It does not mean lying on the sofa with your feet up, mesmerized by the television or radio.

During deep relaxation, refrain from any other activity.

Research has shown that for deep relaxation to be effective, you must have at least one period of relaxation daily, lasting a minimum of fifteen to twenty minutes. Training begins by focusing on breathing and muscle relaxation. But it doesn't matter what form of relaxation you use. What does matter is that you have a consistent and deep experience of relaxation. In such a state, thoughts occur less frequently and do not become fixations. Your breathing becomes slow and regular, and your muscles feel deeply relaxed. This state might be characterized by a heavy, weighty sense of your body, or the opposite—a light, floating sensation. People often report feeling quiet, focused, and passive. All these sensations are usually indications that you're deeply relaxed.

### *Contraction-Release*

One of the most common methods of relaxation is based on the principle of contraction-release in which you tense and then relax successive muscle groups of your body. When tensing a group of muscles, hold them as tightly as possible, then let go and relax completely. Best results are gained through regular practice. If you wish, tape record these instructions, which adds an added self-help element because your own voice is guiding you through the exercise. Also, listening to calming music while doing any of the relaxation exercises can be helpful.

1. Arrange your body in a comfortable, receptive position. Lying on your back on the floor is preferable, but you may sit in a chair if you wish. Uncross your legs and extend your arms along your sides, palms facing up.
2. Take three long, full inhalations, exhaling completely each time. Feel your body let go of tension with each exhalation.
3. Clench your right fist and hold the tension there, tighter and tighter. Study the tension in your right fist as you keep the rest of your body relaxed. Then drop the tension and allow a sensation of relaxation to flow in. Observe the difference between relaxation and tension as a pleasant, heavy feeling floods your hand—into your palm, into each finger.
4. Now, clench your left fist, then release the tension in the same manner as above.
5. Clench both fists and straighten both arms, tensing the

muscles. Hold the tension. Observe the tension. Now release the tension in both arms and let them drop to your sides. Observe the warm, heavy feeling of relaxation flowing into your arms, down the elbows, through the wrists, into the palms. Feel yourself letting go, relaxing. Take a long, deep breath. Exhale slowly, becoming even more relaxed.

6. Take another long, deep breath, filling your lungs. Hold the air in your chest, observing the tension created. Now exhale slowly, observing the walls of your chest loosen as the air is pushed out. Continue relaxing and breathing freely and gently.

7. Tighten your abdominal muscles by pushing them up and out as far as they can go. Hold the tension there and study it. Release the abdominal muscles and allow the feeling of relaxation to flow into each muscle. Continue breathing freely and easily. On each exhalation, notice the pleasant sensation of relaxation spreading throughout your body.

8. Tense your buttocks and thighs by pressing down as hard as you can and by clenching your buttocks muscles together. Hold the tension and study it. Release and allow a deep, soothing feeling of relaxation to flow in.

9. Tense your lower legs by clawing both feet down as hard as you can and pinching your buttocks muscles together. Hold the tension and study it. Release and allow a deep, soothing feeling of relaxation to flow in. Breathe in and out easily and allow relaxation to flow throughout your body.

10. Tense your back and shoulders by pinching your shoulders together and arching your back off the floor. Hold the tension and let go, allowing your back to drop gently back to the floor. Feel the relaxation spread.

11. Roll your head back and forth very gently from side to side, releasing the muscles in the back of your head.

12. Tense your facial muscles by sticking out your tongue as far as it will go, closing your eyes tightly, and wrinkling up your forehead. Hold the tension, then release, allowing warm relaxation to flow through the scalp, forehead, eyelids, cheeks, jaw, even the tongue.

13. Now, allow your body to experience heaviness, as if it's boneless and only the floor is keeping you from sinking. You may, at this time, make a mental inventory of the parts of your body

you have contracted and released, telling yourself as you go through your body that each part is heavy, warm, and relaxed.

14. When you are ready to enter the waking state, begin by gently wriggling toes and fingers, gradually moving into whatever larger stretches your body wants.

15. Roll to one side in a fetal position, place one palm on the ground and push off, lifting your body comfortably and easily into a sitting position.

### *Diaphragmatic Breathing*

A simple form of relaxation involves only the use of the breath. You can use this technique, the Basic Eastern Breath, or Alternate Nostril Breathing to relax you.

1. Relax your entire body as completely as you can. Breathe in through your nose in a natural, easy way.

2. Each time you inhale, feel the breath travel further downward, all the way to the diaphragm, where it loosens those muscles, then all the way to the bottom of your belly, where it loosens the pelvic girdle. Remember to allow your belly to *expand* gently as you take in each breath. Keep your shoulders and chest relaxed and still.

3. Exhale *slowly* through your mouth, emptying the belly, letting your jaw relax and drop. Make each exhalation last as long as possible, but do not hold the breath between inhalations and exhalations.

4. Turn your attention to breathing in and out, slowly, gently, and naturally.

Once you've learned to put yourself in a state of deep relaxation at will, you can simply give yourself an image or word to trigger deep relaxation and you will be completely relaxed. At that point, you will be able to master guided visualization techniques that can greatly improve your sex life.

Start with these simple exercises that combine relaxation with guided visualization:

## RELAXATION/VISUALIZATIONS EXERCISES

These visualizations help to relax and cleanse you—physically and mentally.

### *Energy Flow Visualization*

This visualization is based on the Chinese concept of *chi,* or life energy, discussed in chapter 4. It helps promote the free flow of life-force energy into, through, and out of your body, leaving you feeling more vibrant and sexually alive.

1. Begin, as always, by relaxing your body and breathing deeply and naturally. Do not begin until you feel relaxed.
2. Focus your vision inward. See a golden, sunlit energy streaming through your body, warming you, revitalizing you, energizing you, and cleansing you.
3. Inhale a wave of energy up the front of your body. The wave begins at your toes, and, with each inhalation, moves further toward the top of your head.
4. When the energy reaches the crown of your head, inhale several more times, each time bringing the wave of light from your toes to your head in a single breath.
5. With each exhalation, see this sun energy move down the back of your body, out the back of your heels and into the ground.
6. Now, inhale and circle your entire body with the golden energy. Do this several times.
7. As you watch the energy circle through your body, notice areas of tension and blockage. Direct the golden light into those areas to unblock, release, and soothe them.

   See the golden energy penetrating every cell and fiber, massaging every part of your inner body with warming, purifying radiance. Know that as the light enters your body through the toes, it brings cleansing energy. As it leaves your body through the backs of your heels, it takes along any impurities, tensions, negative thoughts, and worries.
8. When you feel completely relaxed, purified, and revitalized, open your eyes and gently return to the present.

### *Balancing Visualization*

This exercise uses your mind and breath to harmonize your body, bringing it into balance and removing all inhibitions and tensions that obstruct your sexual pleasure.

1. Lie on your back, legs extended about shoulder-width apart, arms extended slightly away from your sides.

2. Inhale a stream of sparkling white light through the sole of your right foot and send it in a diagonal direction across your trunk and all the way down your left arm to your fingertips. Do this until you can send the light all the way through on a single inhalation. Exhale and relax a moment.

3. Inhale the light through the sole of your left foot. Send it diagonally across your trunk and all the way down your right arm, to the fingertips.

4. Do this several times on each side, each time visualizing and feeling life-force energy permeate every cell, giving each cell new life.

5. Now, inhale both diagonal streams of energy through the soles of both feet, crisscrossing and concentrating the energy at your pelvis, then sending it all the way to your fingertips. Do this several times.

6. Visualize a ball of concentrated sparkling white light hovering just over the top of your head. Inhale that energy into your head.

7. Circle it around your brain several times in both directions.

8. Inhale the light down through your body and exhale it out the soles of your feet. Do this several times.

After a few minutes of this exercise, you should feel fully energized, balanced, and relaxed.

### *Purifying Fire Visualization*

This is another effective exercise in which your mind power and breath energize and cleanse your body of physical impurities, muscular tensions, and negative beliefs about your sexuality.

1. Lie on your back, legs extended, about hip-width apart, arms slightly away from your sides.

2. Focus your attention on the crown, or top, of your head.

3. Now, shift your focus to the soles of your feet.

4. Become aware of the space between the crown of your head and the soles of your feet. See that space as an empty container

waiting to be filled and cleansed with the purifying energy of your breath.

5. Inhale deeply through the bottoms of your feet as you visualize pure, white, sparkling life-force energy moving up and filling the container of your body.

6. As the purifying light passes through your body, see all physical impurities and tensions, all fatigue, all negative beliefs and emotions, as dried autumn leaves. The light is gathering up these leaves and carrying them upward.

7. As you exhale slowly and evenly, see the dried leaves exit through your mouth and nostrils then combust in a brilliant flame that incinerates them completely.

8. Keep inhaling the leaves upward and exhaling them into a fiery nothingness, until no more leaves are left, and you are full of sparkling light.

### *Tantric Color Meditation*

Tantric practitioners and increasing numbers of Westerners know that color can exert a powerful effect on our minds and bodies. Scientists have even proven that red stimulates the male reproductive organs, while violet increases the activity of the female sex glands. This exercise uses color to increase the energy and health of your body, especially the sex organs and glands.

1. Sit in a comfortable cross-legged position or in a straight-back chair, making sure your spine is straight and shoulders relaxed.

2. Close your eyes and visualize radiant colors—brilliant rays of red, orange, yellow, green, blue, indigo, and violet—pouring over you in a warm, life-giving flood. Feel each of their luminous energies penetrate every cell and tissue.

3. Relax, letting your entire body go limp for a few moments.

4. Sit upright again and exhale all the air from the lungs, forcing it out by contracting your abdomen.

5. Inhale slowly, expanding your abdomen. Hold your breath for the count of seven, as you visualize the color red (women should substitute violet). See rays of red (or violet) flowing over your lower abdomen and genital area, then see red (or violet) covering the back of your head.

6. Repeat this process three times.

Tantrics advise practicing this color meditation in front of an open window or outdoors in sunlight.

## CREATING YOUR OWN GUIDED VISUALIZATION SCENARIOS

If you can create an imaginary scenario in which you complete every sexual encounter with a blockbuster orgasm, will that image become reality? It's very possible.

Your own guided visualizations are like choreographed daydreams, a script you write, then rehearse until it's ready to become your day-to-day reality. Going over that scripted visualization is like focusing your inner "projector," or your inner "eye," on the inner "movie screen" of your mind.

There's no right or wrong way to do a guided visualization; all that counts is that it produces the results you're after. The degree to which that visualization becomes part of your actual life experience depends, though, on how carefully you create the scenario and how much force of your belief you invest in it.

First, you need to decide precisely and in minute detail what you really want. You may want to write your script—either in your head or on paper—then see how it looks on your inner movie screen, making edits and additions as it plays out.

But beware of answered prayers. Make sure that these images reflect the exact changes that will actually give you greater sexual happiness.

Do you desire a new sexual adventure, to overcome negative feelings about your body, to have multiple orgasms or simultaneous orgasms, or to resolve sexual problems with your partner?

Include in your visualization whatever you think is missing from your sex life. Focus on the vision of you making love with that elusive pleasure in place.

Don't worry whether or not your goal is realistic. The mind can work miracles. Have a little faith and apply a little effort, time, and patience.

If you are self-conscious about your body, you could create a visualization in which you are gloriously nude, dancing gracefully as candlelight flickers over your firm, supple body, and your adoring beloved or a crowd of awed spectators gazes on.

If you are feeling sexually sluggish and your love life is mired in a rut, you could visualize you and your partner—or, if you have no partner, the ideal fantasy partner—making mad, passionate love in new and exciting ways and in strange and exotic locales. You revel in the delights of each other's bodies as you each give and receive fully, then surrender to several simultaneous, heart-pounding orgasms.

If you and your partner are trapped in sexual conflict, you can create a guided visualization to help you become more sensitive, understanding, and empathic with each other.

For example, you could sit opposite each other, close your eyes, and visualize entering each other's body. Then, visualize and feel what it's like to make love as your partner. Speak from his or her perspective, sharing what "you" enjoy, what "you" don't enjoy, and what "you" would like to try.

Switching places gives you insight into what it's like for your partner to be with you and helps overcome misunderstandings and conflicts. In fact, you don't really need to be in conflict to try this visualization; switching places also makes for an exciting sexual adventure.

Amanda stumbled upon this erotic thrill by accident. During an afternoon nap one day, she dreamed that she was her boyfriend making love to herself. She woke up gasping. When a friend asked how it felt, all she could get out was, "Amazing! Amazing!"

### Tips for Creating an Effective Visualization

• Make the images of your visualization as clear, specific, and lifelike as possible.

• Your visualization does not have to conform to the constraints of ordinary reality. It can follow dream logic, where anything goes. You can fly; see sexual desire build in your body as vivid colors, textures, and shapes; become an exotic creature; or enjoy a romance with your favorite movie star.

• Focus not just on your goal, but on how you will get there—the process. For example, you might want to have a vaginal orgasm. See the entire experience: You are enjoying yourself with your partner, perhaps having a romantic dinner. Then, you begin to make love. Don't leave out a single detail and take your time in visualizing each kiss, caress, stroke, every moment of oral sex and intercourse in your favorite positions. See each curve made by your entwined bodies as they heave and sigh in unison. After you've stoked your fires with all the details leading up to your goal, then you can end your imaginary encounter with the full-out fireworks of a mind-bending orgasm. See your body undulate with wave after wave of pure, intense pleasure. Feel every wave.

If your goal is multiple orgasms, see yourself overwhelmed by orgasm after orgasm until you are completely satiated.

If your goal is a simultaneous orgasm with your partner, see the two of you dissolve in mutual rapture.

Involve as many of your senses as possible to make your scenario even more real. Feel, hear, taste—even smell—whatever you're seeing.

Sara achieved a completely successful outcome with her self-scripted visualization. Her goal was to overcome an emotional-sexual problem in which she could relate to a man either sexually or with feelings of love. The problem was that she could never experience both feelings together.

So Sara created a very detailed visualization in which the climactic scene showed a stream of brilliant pink energy making a circle that linked her heart and her pelvis, connecting those centers at the physical, mental, and emotional levels. As she played this image over and over on her inner movie screen, Sara allowed herself to experience a deep longing to merge those two aspects of herself.

Her visualization did become reality, and Sara is now happily married.

- As these images of your sexual desires pass by, sense how each one makes you feel. Do you really want that? Is something else missing from your sex life that needs to be there before you can fulfill that ultimate goal?
- Be aware of all the feelings that arise as you spin out this scenario. Do you feel a yearning, a sweet melting, an excited anticipation, or the calm and sense of completion that comes with ac-

complishing a goal? Is your heart beating faster? Are your palms sweating? Are butterflies dancing in your belly? Is your body all tingly? Is it moving almost involuntarily? Whatever feelings or sensations come up, accept them and experience them fully. They will bring you closer to fulfilling your goal.

• Whenever a particularly appealing image flashes on your inner screen, freeze the frame. Savor that image for a few moments as you tell yourself it's already yours.

• Affirm aloud that you deserve the very best life has to offer, especially a passionate, fulfilling sex life that includes any particular experience you are visualizing.

• Be patient. It may take several trys to get going, and results may not show right away, but they will come. You need time and patience, and remember to welcome any persistent doubts and blocks, because they tell you where you need to go next.

### *How to Deal with Negative Thoughts*

Of course, the less conflicted you are about enjoying a more passionate and fulfilling sex life, the more easily your inner movie will transfer to your real life.

If you are unable to visualize a particular feeling or experience, explore that block and try to discover why you are protecting yourself from that particular sexual experience. Let yourself feel any strong negative feelings associated with that block—fear, anger, anxiety, or irritation. Do not try to suppress them. Ask yourself why you are feeling this way. The answer will tell you what has been blocking your authentic sexuality all along.

Two common negating thoughts are: "I don't deserve sexual pleasure" and "Sex is dirty and I'm dirty if I let myself enjoy it." Do they sound familiar?

Once you uncover your negative thoughts and beliefs, you will realize that you were already playing out a visualization without even knowing it: a negative scenario about your sexuality that fed you an endless loop of sexually defeating suggestions. Don't be afraid to let that movie play out in your mind a few more times, until you can see it clearly as the lie that it is.

Give yourself the same sound counsel you would give a friend. Challenge the validity of your negative thoughts and the feelings they create. Get professional help if necessary, so you can finally overcome these obstacles to your sexual happiness and replace them with more positive beliefs that will create a more fulfilling sexual reality for you.

Remember, you cannot enjoy a new outlook on your sexuality without first cleansing your mind of worn-out, unfulfilling patterns.

Your will and energy are the engine of your visualization, so be open to doing whatever it takes to make it real. Even if you don't entirely believe that a guided visualization can change your sex life, pretend that it will. The power of pretend cannot be undervalued. Over time, pretend develops into the habit of positive thinking and shifts the creations of your imagination into the realm of genuine possibilities.

After you become accomplished in guided visualization techniques, all you will have to do is give yourself a preset signal to relax, then turn your mind briefly to an image or images of what you want in your sex life, and it will be done!

### *Developing Your Imaginative Powers*

You may be saying to yourself, "Sure, that's fine for some, but I have no imagination and my mind constantly wanders. I can't do this!"

Recent research on "guided imagery" does indicate that about 10 percent of people are particularly imaginative, what researchers call "high absorbers." Any sensory stimulation—a piece of music, a beautiful panorama in nature, a whiff of an appealing scent—and their imaginations are so stimulated that they're swept away by a flood of fantasy that packs all the impact of reality.

A high absorber could probably enjoy a fabulous sexual encounter simply by conjuring it up in his or her mind.

The good news is that with practice, you could do that too. We all have a degree of imaginative power, and it can be developed fairly easily.

In fact, if you are practicing any of the breathing, relaxation, and guided imagery exercises you have read about so far, you have already begun to stimulate and enhance your imaginative faculties.

Here's another helpful exercise to develop your imagination:

Read each of the items on the list that follows. See each one as an image in your mind. Take your time. Do this every day for a week. Then, one by one, bring in each of your other senses: smell, taste, touch, hearing. Practice each sense daily for a few days. Stop for a week or so. Then, go over the list, first seeing images of the words, then smelling, tasting, touching, and hearing them.

ITEMS:

your father's face
your unmade bed
a barking dog
a purring kitten
a speeding motorcycle
a stoplight
your favorite chair or sofa
ocean waves lapping at the shore
your best friend
soft fur
a skin rash
your morning shower
jumping as high as you can
brushing your teeth
eating chocolate
coffee percolating (or your favorite tea brewing)
your favorite flower
a child playing

It won't be long before you'll notice how much easier it is for each item to set off a rush of vivid images, sounds, smells, tastes, and feelings. You'll soon realize that you do have a good imagination, after all!

# Part Two

## GREAT SEX, NATURALLY

# 6

# EXPLORING YOUR BODIES

You've reaped the benefits of good nutrition, herbs, supplements, exercises, visualizations, and even special techniques that prepare you for better sex. But in order to truly enjoy great lovemaking, you also need to understand the intricacies of your sexual organs and responses as well as your partner's.

Most of us learn about sex in a haphazard, incomplete fashion, through a patchwork of sources—images on television and in movies, lines from popular songs, and school friends. Only a lucky few get all the right information from open, approachable parents.

Gynecologists across this country report that many of the adults who visit their offices have no idea of what goes where. Even if we know which parts fit together, many of us still do not realize that sex does not begin the moment a man inserts his penis into a woman's vagina. We pay too little attention to foreplay—kissing, touching, stroking, caressing, stimulating each other's genitals—as well as to the role of sexual fantasy and role playing.

The notion that only women enjoy foreplay is one of the biggest sexual misunderstandings that blocks many of us from fulfilling our erotic potential. Men enjoy kissing, touching, licking, hugging, and acting out fantasies just as much as women. As for erotica, women can be as turned on by it as men.

This chapter will teach you how to discover all you need to know about your sexual apparatus and your sexual response. It will answer all your questions about masturbation—solo and mutual—and tell you how to draw every ounce of pleasure from foreplay, intercourse, and orgasm.

# MASTURBATION

Most of our earliest sexual fieldwork involved masturbation. The dictionary defines masturbation as self-stimulation of the genitals for pleasure, but for some of us, masturbation is still the "sin of self-abuse."

Masturbation is actually a harmless pleasure that offers sexual release whenever you need it. It's only a problem when either you or your partner chronically masturbates instead of sharing the sexual experience.

Performed solo, masturbation teaches you about your body. With your partner, it teaches you about your body and your partner's, helping you appreciate both your own and each other's sexuality. Masturbation can even help you gain a surprising degree of control over your sexual response.

Mutual masturbation—watching each other masturbate—can be either an exciting part of foreplay or an end in itself—particularly when birth control isn't handy or when you feel like enjoying a sexy variation on your usual lovemaking themes.

It is also a wonderful way to show what you like in bed, particularly if you are too shy to speak up. If your partner is reluctant or unaware of how to touch you the way you would like, you can do it yourself, while your partner watches.

For instance, if a man believes he should be man enough to satisfy his partner with his penis alone or that only impotent men or men with little penises have to resort to stimulating their partners manually, his partner can tell him that she has something special she wants to share. Her demonstration should turn him on enough to overcome any hesitations or objections.

If the woman is too shy to touch herself in front of her partner, he can help by telling her how exciting it is to him and how sexy and beautiful she looks while doing it.

What does masturbation teach you about?

### *The Clitoris*

The clitoris and the penis are analogues of each other. Both the clitoris and penis are protected by a hood, or foreskin, and both swell with blood and become erect during arousal. In fact, scientists say that we are all female in our early stages in the womb, until male hormones kick in and keep some of us from developing female genitals.

The clitoris measures, on average, about one-sixth of an inch wide and one-sixth of an inch long. The clitoris is actually the tip of a much larger structure located inside a woman's body that also swells during arousal.

Just like penises, clitoral size varies from woman to woman, but has no relationship to capacity for sexual enjoyment. Among the probable determining factors in your sexual enjoyment is how many nerves terminate in and near your clitoris. The greater their density, the greater your sexual thrill.

Some experts also theorize that the ability to orgasm during intercourse is greater if a woman's clitoris is situated closer to her vaginal opening so that the clitoris receives stimulation during the thrusting, bumping, grinding, and winding of intercourse. That may be true for some women, but it's certainly not the case with all women. As we know, the mind is the most powerful sex organ and look how far away it is from the other sex organs!

Most experts agree that the clitoris is nearly twice as sensitive as the vagina, with the upper-left side of the clitoris—from the woman's point of view—being its hot spot. Some women are so sensitive that the pressure of fingers on this area is uncomfortable. So, the guide words for exploring the clitoris are "softly and gently."

### *The Vagina*

Vaginas also come in as many different widths and lengths as penises, with the average vagina measuring about three to four inches from opening to cervix. During intercourse, this shape-changing organ will expand to make room for a large penis, constrict for a thin one, lengthen for a long one, and come forward to accommodate a short one.

The first third of the vagina tends to be more sensitive than the inner two-thirds, and the legendary—and often maddeningly elusive—G-spot is located about two inches up the vagina's front wall.

During adolescence, estrogen levels soar, maturing the vaginal cells and changing the environment from base to acid. During menopause, estrogen levels lower, thereby thinning, drying, and narrowing vaginal walls and shrinking the labia.

When you are sexually aroused, your vaginal walls secrete droplets of lubricating fluid. But yeast infections, sexually transmitted diseases, douching, over-exercising, stress, and menopausal hormonal changes can block lubrication. Some prescription and over-the-counter drugs, including cold and allergy remedies, also dry out vaginal membranes.

If you don't lubricate enough for comfortable masturbation or intercourse, try extending your foreplay. You can also use an unscented, water-soluble lubricant, such as K-Y Jelly, Replens, or Astroglide—all available over the counter. Oil-based lubricants like butter, vegetable oil, or petroleum jelly are not good for the vaginal environment, and they cause the latex in condoms to deteriorate.

The vagina can become overstretched by childbirth, leading to a phenomenon called "tenting," in which the vagina overextends as the penis thrusts in, causing a feeling of slackness for the man. If this has happened to you, you can restore normal tissue tone and strength by practicing Kegel exercises and/or the many other female organ-toning exercises given in chapter 4.

### *The G-spot*

For centuries it was known to Eastern sages as the "sacred spot." We in the West only discovered this extremely sensitive area of the vagina in this century, thanks to Dr. Ernest Grafenberg, for whom we named this tiny erogenous zone. A few years ago, the G-spot was hailed as a discovery on a par with that of the Americas. Indeed, it's an uncharted territory for most Western women, as only 10 percent or so can find this "sacred" part of their anatomy. But once discovered and stimulated, the G-spot is supposed to give a more intense orgasm, which, in some women, is accompanied by a profuse discharge of a clear, sweet liquid that is definitely not urine! The following masturbation tips and the Eastern lovemaking techniques and exercises described in chapter 8 provide guidance, in that they sensitize you to the various aspects of your sexual response.

## HOW TO MASTURBATE SOLO

• Just because you're having a party that only includes "me, myself, and I," doesn't mean you can't set the mood. Turn off the electricity and light a few scented candles. Play soft, sexy music. Watch an erotic video or read erotic literature.

• Don't worry if you find yourself fantasizing about someone other than your partner or someone you wouldn't really want to make love with. Remember, your fantasies do not have to become realities. Enjoy them as harmless flights of fancy.

• Take your time. Make this a full-fledged sexual adventure.

• Use a lubricant (water-based only) or your own saliva.

• Experiment. Some women just squeeze their thighs together, exerting pressure on the clitoris, until they orgasm. Some masturbate on their stomachs, pushing the pelvis into a pillow or towel. Other women prefer to position themselves so that the stream from the bathtub faucet or shower hits their genitals and stimulates them to orgasm.

You can use your fingers to stroke, rub, squeeze, and tickle your inner and outer labia, your clitoris, and to penetrate your vagina.

• You can also use a vibrator or a dildo to stimulate yourself. Some new sex toys vibrate and circle inside the vagina at the same time that they vibrate the clitoris.

Let your imagination roam free and allow it to guide your experiments.

• Try different rhythms, pacing, degrees of pressure, and see what you like best.

• Try stopping just before you climax for a cool-down. Then work yourself back up again. This extends your arousal phase longer and builds it higher, so when you finally do release, you enjoy a longer, stronger orgasm.

## MASTURBATING TOGETHER

Many couples include masturbation in their erotic repertoires, either masturbating each other or doing it in front of each other, even using masturbation to conclude a sensual massage.

### *How to Masturbate Her*

• Always wet your fingers, either with saliva or a lubricant . . . and use a light touch. Be responsive. Check her facial expressions, sounds, and body movements to gauge if she's enjoying what you're doing and exactly which moves she likes best.

• If she has never or rarely orgasmed with you, don't make orgasm your goal. Simply explore and enjoy, with no pressure to perform.

• Vary your movements. Circle the clitoris, move your fingertip or the side of your finger up and down the shaft. A favorite move many women love is to form a V with two fingers and press the juncture of the V just above the clitoris, with the two fingers pressing gently on each side.

• Stimulate the G-spot.

You should both be slightly aroused, and her bladder empty.

As you lie face to face, position your palm up and insert your lubricated index finger and middle finger into her vagina. Push gently against the front vaginal wall as you move upward, until you feel a small patch of rougher skin, usually about one-third of the way up. Your partner's response should confirm whether or not you've struck gold. If you have, stroke the spot by making a come hither gesture with your fingers.

• Stimulate her U-spot.

An even more recent discovery than the G-spot, the U-spot is the opening of the urethral canal, usually located between the clitoris and the vaginal opening.

Not every woman likes this particular button pressed (especially if her bladder is full), so proceed with caution, unless she has already run a few solo tests to see if it turns her on. If she's prone to bladder infections, either skip this spot altogether or make sure your hands are surgery-prep clean.

## HOW TO TEACH HIM

You can show your partner exactly how you like to be pleasured by sitting or lying down, spreading your legs, and then parting your outer vaginal lips so that he can see exactly what you are doing. Demonstrate how you like your inner labia stroked, then spread them apart and show him how you like your clitoris stimulated. Ask him to copy your movements. Then ask him to explore your vagina with his fingers, as you contract and release your PC muscle to increase your excitement.

### *How to Masturbate Him*

- You can use one hand or two, but always wet your hand(s) first. Use your saliva, the lubricating secretion from his penis, or a water-based lubricant.
- Vary your pacing, pressure, and strokes.
- Try the F-spot.

The frenulum is the "scientific" term for the hot spot on the underside of the penis where the head of the penis ends and the shaft begins. Be gentle and don't overdo it, as too much F-spot stimulation can produce a rapid-fire orgasm.

- Try the R-spot.

This spot is really a line, the one that runs along the center of the scrotum and is known as the raphe. The skin of the scrotum is analogous to the sensitive skin on the inner labia.

### How to Teach Her

Cover her hand with yours and show her how to stroke the shaft of your penis to bring you to erection. Guide her hand to the head and the ridge on the underside that joins the head to the shaft and show her how to stroke those especially sensitive areas.

Demonstrate how you like your testicles caressed and how to press on the perineum—the area between the scrotum and anus—and how to fondle the anal opening.

## The Art of Foreplay

First of all, make foreplay fun, not a test of your sexual skills. Second, start making love before you both get naked. Tell each other how much you want each other, exchange long, lingering, steamy looks. Some people are turned on by sexy talk; others prefer action rather than words. Experiment. Share your preferences.

### *Kissing Tips*

Kissing can be incredibly exciting, signaling how much you desire each other and giving the act of sex the ultimate turn-on of romance. Kiss while you're still fully dressed; kiss while you're removing your clothes; kiss after your clothes are all off. Kiss each other everywhere. The ears are particularly sensitive. So is the neck. Explore to find each other's secret spots. Kissing is a wonderful way to express love and desire. It can even foreshadow and mimic the act of intercourse. The right kisses can stoke your heat to incinerating temperatures.

- Make sure your oral hygiene is on point. That means brushing your teeth as well as your tongue. It also means flossing to prevent the build-up of odor-causing plaque and bacteria. If your toothbrush isn't handy when you need oral refreshment, chew gum or suck on a mint.
- Don't go in there as if you're excavating a mine. Start off slowly and lightly—teasing with your lips, nibbling, pressing, rubbing. Your mouth should be only slightly open, lips firm yet supple, covering and cushioning your teeth.
- Go on to licking and sucking your lover's lips. Dart your tongue inside his or her mouth, then pull away for a brief instant and resume those soft kisses.
- When you are both very hot, then you can go for the wide-open, tongue-plunging kisses. Take your cue from your partner. Never force your way in. To the unprepared or unwilling partner, that can feel like oral rape.
- Continue to vary the pace, pressure, and techniques to keep your kissing exciting.
- When you are both very hot, explore your lover's mouth with your tongue, exploring and penetrating every nook and cranny.

### *Touching Tips*

- Run your hands over each other's entire body while you are fully clothed, partially clothed, and after you are naked. Take your time.

• Vary your touching: stroke, knead, and use light, feathery touches.

• This is a great time for verbally sharing how much you are enjoying each other and how excited you are, and for those long, lingering looks.

### *How to Massage Your Lover*

One of the most erotic ways you can touch your partner is to give him or her a love massage.

• Use a small amount of scented oil or lotion—warmed first by your hands. Never dribble oil or lotion over your partner's body like you're dripping mustard on a hot dog.

• Never break contact. Always have at least one hand on your partner's body.

• First, lightly massage your partner from tip to toe, backside first, using a combination of the following strokes:

*Gliding.* Make big, gliding movements that blend into each other all over your partner's skin on the back, chest, breasts, buttocks, and spine.

*Kneading.* This is not the time for deep, painful muscle-release work. Lightly knead your partner's muscles as if you were preparing dough for bread. Special tension-relieving spots include the base of the neck and the shoulders at the top of the back.

*Feathering.* Graze your fingerpads lightly over your partner's skin.

• Use your mouth, hair, breasts, and/or penis, not just your hands, to stroke your partner.

• Knead the buttocks and lightly trail your fingers up and down in between them. You can then stroke the anus and gently massage the perineum.

• After he or she has turned over, use the gliding, kneading, and feathering strokes on the front of your partner's body.

• Glide up and down between the nipples and the genitals.

• Stroke gently and slowly up and down the inner thighs.

• Caress and fondle his or her genitals. Use your partner's response to guide your next moves. You can move to masturbating your partner or performing oral sex. Or you can simply kiss and embrace.

# ORAL SEX

The dictionary defines oral sex as the stimulation of a partner's genitals by mouth or tongue. "Cunnilingus" is the oral stimulation of female genitals, and "fellatio" refers to oral stimulation of male genitals.

Most Americans have given and received oral sex, usually as part of foreplay. In fact, a majority of American women report that oral sex is either the primary or only way they can reach a climax.

However, some men and women still find the prospect of oral sex distasteful. Their concerns center around issues such as taste, smell, and hygiene. This is particularly true of some men who worry that the smell and/or taste of a woman's genitals will turn them off. Yet many more men find the scent and taste of a woman's vaginal juices to be a major turn-on. In fact, men are actually more willing to perform oral sex than most women believe, because women tend to sully the issue with their body image problems.

Some people consider oral sex to be a more intimate and personal act than intercourse. Others feel just the opposite. In any case, one partner's refusal to engage in oral sex can cause serious problems in a relationship.

No one should miss out on this major erotic pleasure. Only the genitals rival the tongue as a perfect bedroom tool. Warm, moist, with a pleasingly rough texture, the tongue can change size and shape and can execute many exciting moves. Several exercises presented a little later in this chapter will increase your tongue's strength, flexibility, and sexual skill. In the case of oral sex, as in so many other of life's activities, practice makes perfect. Communication also helps.

Above all, never forget that if you are inviting someone to dine chez vous, presentation is everything. You must please *all* the senses, and that includes delighting the nose, as well as the eye. Make sure that you're clean and well-groomed. Take a bath or shower together as part of foreplay. You can also apply a tasty edible—water-based—lubricant to your genitals.

### *How to Persuade a Reluctant Partner to Sit at Your Table*

- If your partner is skittish, don't force the issue. Go slowly and gently.
- Be patient with your partner; give him or her enough time to get used to the idea.
- Try to understand the reason for his or her reluctance. It could stem from religious or other social/familial prohibitions, fear of performance failure, problems with anything messy, fear of being turned off, or issues concerning what is manly or womanly.
- Discuss the issue calmly and without judgments. Just getting his or her concerns out in the open and showing understanding can ease those fears and negative fantasies.
- Erotic videos can be instructive and exciting. Watch them together and share your reactions: "Hey, *that* looks like fun!"
- Find a position that is comfortable for you both, physically and psychologically. Let the reluctant lover choose the position.
- Use positive reinforcement when he or she does finally do the deed: "Are you sure this was the first time you ever did this?"

## HOW TO PERFORM CUNNILINGUS

Make sure both of you are comfortable. Some good positions: She lies on her back with her legs drawn up and spread. You lay between her legs, your arms under her legs and your hands supporting and caressing her buttocks. You can also tuck a pillow under her buttocks so that her labia opens wider and her clitoris protrudes. Or, you can lie on your back, while she kneels and straddles your face.

Start out slowly and gently, and don't go straight for her genitals. Draw out the excitement of her anticipation. Kiss her inner thighs, massage her stomach, stroke her labia lightly.

Monitor your partner's reactions. Her movements, how she grips your body, her sighs, moans, rapid breathing, and other signs will guide you as to what feels good to her and what doesn't.

Lick the entire genitalia with long, slow strokes. Part the outer vaginal lips, then use your tongue to stroke the inner lips.

Experiment with different oral strokes, pressure, and pacing to find what feels good to her. Flick, tickle, lick, suck, and press.

Don't be afraid to follow any inspiration, remembering to pay close attention to her reactions in order to gauge her pleasure. If something doesn't seem to turn her on, stop and try something else.

Do not move to the clitoris until she is wet with vaginal juices and the clitoris is erect. You can also add your own saliva. Don't use too much pressure, as this is a highly sensitive, nerve-rich area. Too much pressure or too much time in one spot can transform stimulation into irritation. While the upper-left side of the clitoris—from her point of view!—is usually especially sensitive, the underside can be sensitive to the point of painful.

Use your tongue to circle the clitoral tip. Run it up and down the shaft. Flick your tongue across the tip of the clitoris and the shaft. Suck the clitoris and labia with your lips, but, remember, easy does it. Use your tongue to probe and lick the inside of her vagina. This last move makes a great segue from oral sex to intercourse. As always, be creative.

A thirty-something bank executive named Carol especially loves when her boyfriend "writes" the alphabet on and around her clitoris. Or you could write the numbers, counting from one to one hundred . . . slowly.

If she begins moving her pelvis, adapt the rhythms of your tongue movements to hers. Use your hands along with your tongue and lips. Stimulate her vagina with your fingers or gently stroke and squeeze her thighs and buttocks while you lick her clitoris.

Some women love the vibrating sensation created when a man hums as he works. But never blow air into the vagina. Air bubbles can enter the bloodstream and even cause a fatal embolism.

### *Receiving Cunnilingus*

Just because you're on the receiving end doesn't mean that you just have to lie there and take it. You can ratchet up the excitement with the following moves:

Contract your anal and PC muscles now and then. This sends a surge of sexual energy to your genitals and gives your vaginal lips an enticing pout. Also, show him where you want him and how much pressure he should give you with a gentle guiding hand on his head. Moan, sigh, and move your hips in time to his movements when he's doing it right, so he receives that all-important positive reinforcement.

## HOW TO PERFORM FELLATIO

If your partner's nipples are sensitive, start off by licking and sucking his nipples, then kiss, nibble, and lick your way down to his genitals. Softly stroke and fondle his penis and scrotum with your hands.

Make sure both of you are comfortable. The 69 position (mouth to genitals) is best for deep throating, but you have more control if he's lying on his back, while you kneel at a right angle to his hip.

Begin by lightly flicking the head of the penis with your tongue tip. Flick up and down the shaft, then switch to longer, more lingering strokes with a bit more pressure. Swirl your tongue around the head of the penis. Stretch your lips so they cover your teeth, then suck the head of the penis. Swirl your tongue around the ridge as you suck.

Take his penis deeply into your mouth, then work your throat muscles in a swallowing movement that stimulates the head of his penis. At the same time, use your tongue to make long slow strokes up and down the shaft. If you're *really* coordinated, you can also cradle and fondle his scrotum with a free hand.

In another interesting scenario, run the tip of your tongue along the ridge under the penis head as you circle the base of his penis firmly with two fingers. Then, lick the head and shaft.

Try alternating deep throating with taking in just the head. Seventies porn star Linda Lovelace built a lucrative career on the strength of her deep-throat talents. It's not all that difficult. The key is in making sure that your throat and mouth are not at a right angle to your neck and in remembering to breathe through your nose. (That should be easy after doing those Eastern breathing exercises.)

Again, your best position for this alignment is 69, with you on your side. Over time, your gag reflex will subdue, and fellatio will become more comfortable.

Vary your tonguing styles, suction, rhythm, speed, and pressure. Take your cues from his responses.

Take brief breaks to let his arousal subside. Kiss his scrotum, thighs, and abdomen. Many men love long, slow licks on the nipples and along the border between the inner thigh and the scrotum. Then, go back to directly stimulating his penis.

Use your hand to caress his testicles or rub up and down his shaft while you orally stimulate the head. Don't be afraid to exert pressure. The general rule is to go firmer than you think you should.

### *Receiving Fellatio*

Don't force your penis into her mouth or thrust too hard. Also, don't be a silent macho man. Release those moans, groans, and sighs of pleasure; wriggle your hips and let her know in any other verbal or nonverbal way how much she's turning you on and how much you appreciate it.

## TAOIST TONGUE LOVE

Taoists view the tongue as a sex organ. That is, like the genitals, it is a major conduit for the exchange of sexual energy. Oral sex parallels and mimics not only penile-vaginal intercourse, but deep kissing. According to Taoists, the thrill of all these activities comes from the merging and exchanging of sexual energy.

A nimble, powerful tongue is like a magic wand that sets off sparks of intense pleasure wherever it touches. Here are a few exercises (adapted from *Taoist Secrets of Love: Cultivating Male Sexual Energy* by Mantak Chia and Michael Winn) to give your tongue extra sparks. Once you get over the giggles and apply yourself, these unusual exercises will give your tongue virtuoso bedroom skills.

### *Lifts and Swings*

#### VARIATION ONE

1. Thread through the center of an orange or apple with a string and secure one end of the string so that the fruit hangs a

few inches in front of and away from your mouth. You can also use a child's rubber ball.

2. Dart your tongue straight out like a snake, making sure the tip touches the fruit with firm pressure. Keep your tongue stiff and straight and try to establish an even rhythm. Over time, work your way up to a faster and faster pace without losing the steady rhythm.

This move is great on nipples, the tip of genitals, even on the inside of the ear.

### Variation Two

Stretch your tongue down to your chin, then move it forward, so that you hook and lift the bottom of the orange or apple on your tongue.

This is a great G-spot stimulating move.

### Variation Three

Stick your tongue out and make it rigid. Swing it all the way to the left, then, as fast as you can, to the right so that it slaps the fruit. Keep slapping the fruit back and forth with ever-increasing force.

This exercise increases oral strength and dexterity, and is especially good for stimulating the penis.

Knock yourself out with these fruit exercises. Pretend you're an N.B.A. player and dribble the fruit, catching it on your tongue tip, sides, and top, balancing and perhaps even twirling it.

When you're a pro with the apple or orange, move up to a grapefruit.

### *Tongue Power Lifts*

1. Hold a ruler a few inches from your mouth.

2. Use the base of your tongue to lift up, then depress the ruler. You can exert a little pressure in the opposite direction, using the hand that's holding the ruler. These power lifts will give your tongue a body builder's strength.

# 7

# UNDERSTANDING ORGASM

The orgasm has been a major focus of attention in nearly every culture throughout recorded history. From the time tantric yogis and Taoists first applied themselves to the subject over five thousand years ago, right up to today's sex researchers and therapists, numerous strategies have been offered to delay male orgasm; ensure, accelerate, and multiply female orgasm; and help men and women share several orgasms simultaneously.

After millions, perhaps billions, of words have been written on this perennially fascinating topic, the orgasm is still shrouded in mystery.

The subject is also so obscured by misinformation and emotion that before we can discuss how to achieve or enhance an orgasm, we have to first understand exactly what it is and how your own concepts of orgasm can be inhibiting.

For men—unless under the influence of a prescription drug that depresses libido and sexual performance (such as an antidepressant) or suffering from certain physical ailments, such as prostatitis or cardiovascular disease—an orgasm is almost a certainty.

For most women, though, it is a sometime event. For a smaller percentage of American women, it never happens at all. According to *The Hite Report,* only 52 percent of sexually active American women—not women in general—have orgasms regularly, either by penile-vaginal intercourse or by manual or oral stimulation.

Yet the female orgasm is the yardstick against which a sexual encounter is generally measured. The female orgasm has become more than a pleasure. It is a validation of a woman's sexuality: "Will I have an orgasm? If I don't, am I a real woman?"

Conversely, a man is a good lover if he "gives" his partner an orgasm, preferably more than one, every time they make love. That goal can provoke the two primary male sexual concerns: fear of ejaculating, or coming, "too soon" and not being able to achieve and/or sustain an erection.

Male orgasm may be even more misunderstood. Many men—and women too—confuse ejaculation with orgasm. What many of us fail to realize is that just because a man has ejaculated does not mean he is realizing his full orgiastic potential.

In other words, men need just as much help as do women in fulfilling their true orgasmic potential.

While the pressure is on for both men and women, the good news is that true sexual fulfillment is possible for virtually everyone. Any woman can have an orgasm, especially if she has used the excellent preparatory techniques described in previous chapters.

There's even better news: though most women need manual or oral clitoral stimulation to have an orgasm, a few simple techniques enable almost anyone to enjoy orgasm from intercourse alone—if you choose to do so. And men can learn how to transform mere release into a powerful, all-consuming flight to the stars.

## What Is Orgasm?

The French call it *le petit mort*, meaning, the little death. The roots of the word orgasm include the Greek *orgasmos*, meaning to grow ripe, swell, be lustful, and the Sanskrit *urja*, meaning nourishment and power.

Above all, the orgasm is one of life's rare and exquisite pleasures: it costs absolutely nothing and isn't even fattening. It is your birthright, but it's not your goal.

## The Female Orgasm

Physiologically, a woman's orgasm occurs only after she has reached her peak of sexual excitement, which means that her clitoris and vagina are completely swollen with blood. Orgasmic release consists of a series of rhythmic spasms of the vagina (and sometimes the uterus) that are triggered by this physical and psychological stimulation. It usually lasts three to twenty seconds, with intervals of less than a second between the first three to six contractions. When an orgasm is really powerful, the entire musculature engages in these rhythmic spasms. After orgasm, the blood that has engorged her genitalia ebbs away.

Of course, a woman's orgasm can feel like so much more.

Orgasm during intercourse is one of Mother Nature's perfect plans: Her way of ensuring that the female retains as much sperm as possible so that conception is more likely to occur and the species will survive. One study has found that if a woman climaxes any time between one minute before to forty-five minutes after her partner ejaculates, her vaginal contractions help her draw up and retain much more ejaculate than if she doesn't orgasm at all.

### *What Percentage of Women Do Orgasm?*

Most studies also agree that between 10 and 15 percent of American women never reach orgasm at all, even through masturbation. These studies also find that only 30 or so percent of women experience orgasm by penetration alone. And most of those women report that their orgasms during intercourse are much less intense than the ones they have from masturbation or oral sex. A lucky 10 percent or so of women climax from kissing, having their breasts licked and sucked, or their thighs stroked or licked. An even smaller percentage need only a nuzzle on the neck or ears to explode, and a very select few orgasm during sleep, waking up from an erotic dream just as they are climaxing. I've even heard that one or two women in this world can simply think themselves to orgasm.

### *Why Are Some Women More Orgasmic Than Others?*

It should come as no surprise to learn that the second most common sexual complaint made by American women—just behind lagging libido—is the inability to orgasm during intercourse.

At least one major reason for the inability to orgasm, to orgasm during intercourse, or simply have the intensely satisfying orgasms most women crave, is lack of sexual desire. And the major causes of low libido are poor nutrition, insufficient rest, and lack of exercise.

Some sex pundits also blame anatomy. Their theories involve

clitoral position and size. For example, if the clitoris is large or positioned so that the shaft of the penis strokes the clitoral region during intercourse, the woman is more likely to orgasm. Much more plausible are those theories that claim if a woman aligns herself just the right way with her partner's body and moves her hips just the right way, she will get the clitoral stimulation she needs to climax.

Sabine, a divorced French woman in her late forties living in Southern California, was frustrated by the lack of a discernible pattern in her orgasms. She always had them when she masturbated. Sometimes she had them during intercourse with a man; other times she didn't. It didn't seem to have much to do with her feelings toward the man, so she began to suspect that the determining factor was anatomical compatibility.

Once she began deliberately experimenting with different positions, even with very subtle shifts of her body position, she found she was able to enjoy more orgasms more regularly.

But even "position" theories don't explain why some women orgasm in positions where the clitoris cannot possibly be stimulated through intercourse, such as the man entering from the rear or "doggy style."

In the main, most experts agree that among the most probable factors that determine whether or not you have an orgasm, and how, have to do with psychology. Do you feel entitled to sexual pleasure? Are you comfortable with your body? Do you enjoy the kind of free sexual thoughts and fantasies that enhance a sexual experience? Does viewing your partner's face and allowing him to view yours during intercourse excite you or would you rather not look?

Of course, if you suffered sexual abuse as a youngster, or your first sexual experience was unpleasant or traumatic, you're naturally less likely to enjoy sex, let alone allow yourself the total release and surrender of orgasm. If this is your situation, an understanding partner and a good professional counselor can help you overcome the fears and blocks created by your past experience.

The quality of your relationship must be figured into the equation. Loving and trusting your partner may not guarantee orgasms, but it helps. Plus, you are more likely to share your concerns and experiment and learn together.

Theresa, an African-American woman in her thirties, never had orgasms, except when she masturbated alone. It wasn't until her late twenties, when she met her future husband, the love of her life, that Theresa suddenly discovered orgasms during love-making. In fact, the chemistry between them was so combustible that Theresa soon was having orgasm after orgasm during intercourse, with no direct clitoral stimulation at all.

Lorie, a hat designer in her fifties who is twice divorced, says, "I never orgasmed with my first husband. I had some orgasms with my second husband, because our relationship was so emotional. My current boyfriend, whom I'm crazy about, just touches me and I'm ready to go off!"

Happily, many women become more orgasmic as they get older. The confidence and sense of self that often graces one's thirties, forties, and beyond leads to a more relaxed attitude and a willingness to let go. The thirties especially are also a time when your hormones are more balanced and humming, so sexual desire runs high, which often leads to more intense and frequent orgasms.

### *Vaginal Versus Clitoral*

Perhaps this country's biggest sexual controversy surrounds the subject of clitoral versus vaginal orgasms. In the sixties, William H. Masters and Virginia Johnson came up with a "scientific" method of measuring the physiological events of female orgasm. At the same time, the second major battle of this century for women's rights was brewing. A debate has raged ever since. Are vaginal and clitoral orgasms the same or are they different? Is one better than the other?

Until the sixties, prevailing wisdom adhered to Freud's notion that "immature" women have clitoral orgasms, while "mature" women experience vaginal orgasms. In *Three Essays on the Theory of Sexuality,* Freud wrote that when little girls become women, they "change their leading erotogenic zone" from the clitoris to the vagina, and "if they fail to do so, they'll be prone to neurosis and hysteria."

Along come Masters and Johnson and the women's liberation movement. Masters and Johnson hooked women up to machines and measured the physiology of female sexual response. In their landmark sex tome, *Human Sexual Response,* they reported that there was no difference between vaginal and clitoral orgasms, after all. In fact, orgasms, they contended, are achieved through the clitoris, and the clitoris alone. This "scientific" evidence, along with Anne Koedt's *The Myth of the Vaginal Orgasm* and Susan Lydon's *The Politics of Orgasm,* challenged the Father of Psychoanalysis and exploded his "myth." The clitoris became the focal point as well as the engine that drives all female orgasms. Feminists added a political element that bolstered the "scientific" findings by contending that the myth of vaginal orgasm had been created by men in order to keep women enslaved to their penises, and, by extension, dependent on them. Now, women were free to pleasure themselves and each other.

The end result is that for three decades or so, the vagina has played second fiddle to its more celebrated neighbor.

If the sexual experience is viewed from a strictly physiological approach, if it is an event that actually can be measured by electrodes and pictured on a graph, then, yes, orgasms are alike, be they vaginal or clitoral in origin.

But a sexual experience adds up to more than the sum of its moving genital parts, and this is one human function that clearly transcends physiology. Ultimately, the orgasm is an intensely subjective, personal experience that eludes our finest, most persistent scientific efforts to contain and define it.

Of course, there's no right or wrong way to have an orgasm. But since no two orgasms are the same, some *must be* better than others! Masters and Johnson notwithstanding, many women—too many to count—are coming out of the closet to state unequivocably that vaginal orgasms are better than clitoral, because they are more profound, powerful, satisfying, and complete.

The expression "earth-moving" comes to mind. When a woman opens her body and invites a man to enter her, she is allowing him to penetrate her deepest self. And when each of them orgasm within the context of this extreme, "plugged-in" intimacy, an explosive energy moves through them both. They are swept up in ripples of mutual pleasure that cannot be measured and charted by any machine. After it's over, both lovers feel whole and grounded, at peace. Poets have attempted in vain to describe this wonderfully ineffable sensation, so how could it be reduced to pat scientific theories or neat categories?

Nevertheless, a vaginal orgasm is not a measure of your worth as a woman, nor should it be your goal. It is, though, a pleasure you deserve.

### *Faking Orgasms*

Most women have faked an orgasm at one time or another. They lie either to protect their partner's ego, because they want to terminate a less than exciting sexual encounter, or because they want to avoid a long postcoital discussion about why they didn't climax.

An occasional faked orgasm to stop an encounter politely without hurting your partner's feelings is one of life's little courtesies. Chronic faking is another story. If you are constantly faking it, you are depriving yourself. If you are not having orgasms, you need to let your partner know how he can help.

The information and guidance you have received so far and everything you will discover in this chapter will help you have any kind of orgasm you want, including vaginal orgasms. And if you are not satisfied with the frequency and intensity of the orgasms you're already having, the same techniques will make them better. Whether you want to have vaginal orgasms, multiple orgasms, or simultaneous orgasms with your partner, the information you need is here.

## HOW TO BECOME ORGASMIC AND HOW TO HAVE MORE AND BETTER ORGASMS

### *Masturbate*

If you've never orgasmed, this is your surest route to the Big O. Whatever you learn about your body through your solo personal experience can then be communicated to your partner.

During intercourse, you can also try manually stimulating your clitoris and the outside of your labia or vulva, or asking your partner to stimulate you with his hand.

### *Tease Yourself*

Don't go straight for the genitals. Take the scenic route. Instead of intensely pursuing an orgasm, let your desire build to a level right before you peak. Then lessen your stimulation so you can hover at that brink for as long as you can without falling over. If you need to, call a brief time-out so your arousal level subsides a little. Move to a less sensitive area for a few minutes. Then, build the excitement back up again.

The more sexual tension you gather, cool down, then gather again, the more likely your orgasmic release and the sweeter it will feel. Savor the maddening pleasures of this sexual roller coaster. Build up and back off a few times, and when you actually let yourself go, it will be outrageous, a head-to-toe burst of total pleasure. You can do this alone, with your partner, or teach him how to do it to you.

Teasing is also a good way to have an orgasm through intercourse. Build up to the boiling point by your usual means, then switch to intercourse just before your orgasm.

### *Free Your Mind*

Don't let negative, fearful thoughts and beliefs distract you from being in the moment. If you think, "I can't climax" or obsess on any other variations on that theme in the middle of making love, it definitely won't happen.

Worry and tension have an actual physiological effect as well: they cut down the blood circulation to your vagina that you need for full arousal and a really good orgasm.

Do whatever you can to ease your anxiety. If you're self-conscious about your body, turn off the lights and use a few candles. Wear sexy lingerie that covers any body areas that trouble you. Focus all your attention on receiving pleasure. Don't let any other concerns get in your way.

Don't obsess about orgasms. You'll wind up feeding yourself an endless loop of negative suggestions, and you'll make it even harder to climax. Instead, focus on the sensuality of the entire experience. Take a page from the *Kama Sutra* and other Eastern sex guides. Westerners tend to treat sex as a sporting event at which we must excel and score. Eastern sex is more about being in the moment—a goalless, blissful state of sexual arousal, in which you have nowhere to go but even higher. If you often find yourself approaching but never actually climaxing, release your expectations and enjoy the present moment.

### *Ditch the Guilt*

Don't feel guilty about enjoying sex. Forget what anyone else has told you. You may have internalized someone else's ideas, like, "It's perverted to masturbate, to enjoy sex with someone, and to have orgasms." It isn't.

### *Show and Tell*

If you know what turns you on, don't be afraid to show and/or tell your partner. You did not come with a set of instructions, so he's probably in the dark—figuratively, that is—about exactly how to please you and what he can do to help you have a great orgasm. Chapter 6 gave you tips on how to show your partner what you like. If you're not shy, you can tell him outright: "I like it best when you stroke me that way," and so on.

Don't limit your erotic possibilities by confining sexual thoughts to when you're actually making love. You're not likely to get wild and be satisfied if your mind doesn't turn to the subject of lovemaking now and again.

Indulge your romantic and sensual side. Dream about your ideal lover. Read a good "bodice ripper," that is, a romance novel, even if you think they're silly. Wear sexy underwear and douse yourself in delicious scents. Take long, lingering, candlelit baths scented by fragrant essential oils and let your mind wander.

Test out sex toys, watch X-rated videos, talk dirty to yourself, act out a fantasy, read erotic literature. Get a head start; by the time you get together with your lover, you'll be more than ready.

### *Deny Thyself*

An occasional period of sexual abstinence gives you time to replenish your hormone supply and puts you in a chronic state of extreme sexual desire. The neurotransmitter dopamine and the hormone testosterone are key players in sexual arousal and excitement. Allow a few days or so for your body levels of these erotic chemicals to rise, and your pay-off will be supercharged orgasms.

### *Find That G-spot*

If you can locate it, your G-spot is said to be as close to a magic orgasm button as you'll ever find. See chapter 6 for directions.

Keep in mind that we each have our ideas about what feels good. If pressing on the G-spot doesn't make the earth move, move on.

If it does prove arousing, here's a technique either you or your partner can use: Manually or orally, touch both the clitoral tip and the U-spot at the same time that pressure is applied to the G-spot.

### *Stay in Sync*

If you and your partner are in sync, that is, if your pace and rhythms match, you should glide together to orgasmic bliss. This is true whether you are stimulating each other manually, orally, or through intercourse.

### *Use Your Mind Power*

A longer, more intense orgasm, full of peaks of pleasure, is a lot more fun than the usual quick release. To have a deeper, longer-lasting orgasm, stop moving just before your climax and visualize the sexual energy building in your genitals, then shooting up your spine and into every cell of your body.

### *Master Kegeling*

Kegels and the sex-enhancing preparatory exercises of chapters 4 and 5 will give you the tone and sensitivity that make orgasms inevitable. Follow the advice in the first three chapters on diet, herbs, and supplements to ensure your sexual health and energy. The depth of sensation and control over your sexual response that you will gain practically guarantees that you will orgasm whenever and however you wish.

### *Practice, Practice, Practice*

Practice whatever works for you—with your partner or without, using genitals, hands, tongue, or lips—until it's perfect.

## HOW TO HAVE A VAGINAL ORGASM

The story of a thirty-year-old college professor who climaxed only from clitoral stimulation sheds light on this controversial subject. When she was told by her bioenergetic psychotherapist that she could be experiencing vaginal orgasms and that they would help integrate her considerable store of energy and reduce her panic attacks, she was initially defensive.

Grudgingly, she followed the therapist's advice: to avoid clitoral stimulation during sex and begin with the female on top position. She also had therapy sessions in which she learned and practiced the bioenergetic exercises in chapter 5 in order to release long-held muscular tensions in the pelvic and abdominal regions and to deepen her breathing.

"Over the course of weeks, I actually felt the focus of sexual excitement move from my clitoris down toward my vagina," she reported to her therapist. "Gradually, that energy moved deeper into my vagina, so that I finally became most orgasmic when my boyfriend was on top. I began having multiple orgasms, and then simultaneous orgasms, and, no matter how many orgasms I had, my boyfriend's climax would trigger my own."

Virtually every suggestion and exercise in this chapter and all the previous chapters will help you have vaginal orgasms. Here are more tips:

### *Get a Grip*

Toning your PC muscle through Kegeling and Eastern exercises gives you stronger orgasms, and a stronger love muscle will help you orgasm, even if you never had one before. Contracting and squeezing your PC muscles stimulates you more and increases lubrication, all of which bring on orgasm. And when you practice these "pelvic push-ups" during intercourse, you can easily build yourself up to the point of an intense vaginal orgasm.

### *Experiment with Positions*

Remember that most of the clitoral nerve structure is internal. Experiment to find intercourse positions that put pressure on the vaginal-urethral-clitoral area termed by some sex researchers "the orgasmic crescent." You don't necessarily have to be touched directly to climax. The right position can add diffuse pressure from your partner's pelvis or belly to the stimulation of vaginal-penile intercourse and bring you to climax.

### *Get on Top*

As seen in the case of the professor described above, the female superior position can be a great "first" position that enables you to "learn how to orgasm" during intercourse. Some women prefer it all the time because it allows them to control angle and depth of penetration, as well as speed of movement. For added clitoral friction, lower your torso so it's snug against his torso, tighten your legs, and rock your pelvis against his.

### *Try Ole Mish*

Not so long ago, it seemed every movie featured a woman roughriding her man. The underlying message? Woman-on-top is for today's strong, passionate women. Ole mish, on the other hand, is for . . . missionaries.

Yet this position is my personal favorite, and one of my life's missions is to rehabilitate this classic from its current and undeserved rep as boring and unimaginative.

Actually, the man-on-top is the most likely position in which a woman will have a vaginal orgasm. Human females are unique in that their vaginas tilt forward, another neat example of biology as sexual destiny. This feature means that face-to-face intercourse is natural and comfortable, and sex has become associated with intimacy and love between the partners. As a young man once noted, "This is the position I use when I'm in love."

You may discover that the missionary position offers you the closest genital and emotional contact. The woman's "orgasmic crescent" is stimulated, and the man is able to thrust his penis deeply. An orgasm in this position can be the most profoundly exciting and satisfying orgasm of all.

## HOW TO HAVE MULTIPLE ORGASMS

Multiple orgasms occur when a woman (or a man) has a second, third, or more orgasms without completely returning to the resolution phase, during which sexual tension and arousal are dramatically reduced.

Sexologists generally agree that all women are capable of having multiple orgasms, but fewer than 50 percent ever do. Men are supposedly not able to enjoy multiples, because each male orgasm is followed by a resolution phase. Women don't require that physical recovery time to jump from one orgasmic peak to another.

Orgasms are not about numbers. More is not necessarily better, because you can get as much emotional and physical pleasure from one orgasm as a dozen. And too many strong orgasms can actually be weakening.

Susan's boyfriend was thrilled by her multiple orgasms. Since he thought they reflected on his prowess as a lover, he worked to "give" her as many as possible and would tally the total for each sexual encounter.

Eventually, Susan began to feel a sensation of weakness and emptiness in her uterus that soon led to persistent inflammation. The condition baffled her gynecologist. It wasn't until she visited a noted Chinese acupuncturist-herbalist that she was told her condition was caused by "not too much sex, but too strong sex."

The tantric and Taoist exercises in chapter 4 and the tantric and Taoist lovemaking techniques in chapter 8 allow you to experience many powerful orgasms without exhausting yourself and endangering your health. In fact, these orgasms increase your sexual energy and overall vitality.

Here are tips to help you enjoy yourself multiply:

### *Use Your Mind Power*

Think "multiple" and that mental preparation will eventually make "more than one" your reality.

### *Start with Oral Sex*

Some women have an orgasm by oral stimulation first, after which they find it easier to have an orgasm through intercourse.

On the other hand, Melanie, a twenty-something airline attendant, found that if she had an orgasm from oral stimulation, vaginal intercourse was actually a little painful. If she switched from oral stimulation to intercourse at the moment just before her climax, then she'd have a more intense orgasm, even two.

### *Ride the Roller Coaster*

The same techniques for intensifying orgasms can also give you multiples. After you've orgasmed, let your stimulation level drop off slightly, then use a lighter, teasing touch to maintain a low-level arousal, waiting a while before you increase stimulation and build up to another orgasm.

## The Male Orgasm

Few men are willing to confess their sexual naiveté. Most men learn about sex through masturbation—the goal of which is "to get off," that is, have an orgasm as speedily as possible. That translates into the sad truism that many men do not know enough about how to make love.

Lack of sexual knowledge is another reason why many men mistakenly believe that ejaculation is all there is to orgasm, and that unlike women, they can orgasm only once per sexual encounter. Contrary to popular wisdom, men can be almost as multi-orgasmic as women.

The key to understanding male orgasm is to recognize that ejaculation is a separate event from orgasm. Through various techniques—most of which you know from chapter 4, as well as those you will learn in chapter 8—a man can develop enough control to postpone ejaculation indefinitely, while enjoying several orgasms and even using those orgasms to heal and revitalize himself and/or his partner.

All this may seem impossibly esoteric and far-fetched, but it's very real and very possible. Instead of being subject to the whims of your penis and having to settle for the usual genital-centered release, you can have sex for as long as you wish and then surrender to the far more intense and rejuvenating experience of one or more "whole-body orgasms."

Even if you're satisfied with the orgasms you're having, like many men, you may reach orgasm more quickly during lovemaking than you or your partner would like.

The following suggestions and techniques will help you to delay your orgasm, experience multiple orgasms, and enjoy more intense, longer-lasting orgasms.

The foundation skill of all these techniques is being able to sense when you are about to come and having enough control to hold back that urge. Instead of discharging orgasmic energy through your penis, you "pump" that energy up your spine to the crown of your head by practicing the Taoist Energy Transformation exercise described in chapter 4. Then, if you wish to use that energy to heal and energize, you can direct the energy flow down the front of your torso so that it makes a complete circuit of your body.

## HOW TO DELAY MALE ORGASM

### *Vary Your Thrusting Pattern*

Alternate deep thrusts during intercourse with shallow ones. When you feel yourself hovering at the brink of orgasm, stop thrusting and remain still within your partner for several seconds or however long it takes for that sensation to subside.

### *Use the Perineum Press*

This ancient Taoist technique is simple but effective. Just before you reach the point of no return, press the tips of three fingers against the perineum, the area between the scrotum and the anus. Practice first while you're masturbating, to make sure you've got the right spot and you're applying enough pressure.

### *Contract Your PC Muscles*

Here's where all that Kegeling and those tantric and Taoist exercises come in especially handy. Just when you're about to orgasm, stop moving and pull out so that you're barely penetrating your partner's vagina. Do not pull out completely. Relax, then do a Kegel squeeze. Hold for a few moments, then resume shallow thrusting strokes.

### *Alternate Stimuli*

Again, just as you're about to peak and explode, stop whatever you're doing and switch to something that will stimulate you less and delay your orgasm.

## HOW MEN CAN EXPERIENCE MULTIPLE ORGASMS

The same techniques that allow you to prolong sex and intensify your orgasm also allow you to experience half a dozen or more orgasms, without ejaculating or losing your erection. You will experience all the sensations of orgasm, although the sensation will be less sharp and focused and more generalized and diffuse. As you can see, the primary requisite for multiple orgasms in men is toned PC muscles.

### *Activate the Perineum Press*

Use the perineum press described above as often as you need to. This technique can do more than prolong your orgasm. After delaying ejaculation several times, you feel as if you've orgasmed without ejaculating.

### *Practice the Exercises in Chapter 4*

Once you can perform the Taoist Energy Transformation exercise on your own, you can do it with a partner and enjoy several powerful orgasms without ejaculating.

## How to Have Simultaneous Orgasms

### *For Her*

#### Get a Head Start

Most women take a bit longer to get warmed up, so you may have to level the playing field by starting before him. If you are going to make love in the evening, prime yourself by thinking sexy thoughts and/or reading or viewing something erotic beforehand. If you're together for a while before making love, think about what you're going to be doing to each other later. By the time you begin making love, you'll be ready.

#### Let Him Help You Get a Head Start

Ask your lover to take his time stimulating you during foreplay. Tell him that you want to savor the experience fully and for as long as possible.

### *For Him*

Since men tend to climax before women, practice any of the above techniques for delaying orgasm. Your partner can help by masturbating you, stopping just before you come, and using the perineum press herself or stopping her strokes, until your excitement level subsides a little. Then she resumes her strokes and brings you up again. You can do this several times together to get used to riding the arousal roller coaster.

### *For Both of You*

#### Practice the Taoist Exercises in Chapter 4

With the degree of strength and control you'll both have, you can work sexual wonders together.

#### Stop His Orgasm

If the man is close to orgasm, either of you can squeeze the base of his penis for a few seconds or use the perineum press, or he can do a long Kegel squeeze.

#### Vary Thrusting Patterns

Whether or not a woman has a vaginal orgasm or a man has a powerful orgasm has a lot to do with the flexibility of their pelvises—that is, their ability to "wind their waistlines" and vary their movements. The man can push in deeply while both partners rotate their hips in unison, "grinding" against each other in a circular motion. You can alternate circular grinds and winds with rapid and vigorous thrusts and with smooth, even strokes; deep penetration with more shallow penetration.

#### Vary Your Pace

Speed up and slow down. Varying the speed, like varying thrusting patterns, prolongs and intensifies the experience.

### Pause

An occasional pause allows both of you to savor the sensations of penetration and cool down a bit.

### Take Breaks to Make Love in Different Ways

Again, variety adds spice and allows you to tease and play with your arousal levels.

### Change Positions Several Times

Experimenting with different positions changes the dynamics and adds variety to lovemaking. Some positions enhance stimulation in different areas of the genitals, thus bringing you more in sync with each other. Some positions are simply more comfortable for your individual body structures or physical conditions. Changing positions during intercourse also breaks up the action for a few moments and helps delay his orgasm, until she is ready to climax herself. It also helps to find the position that allows you both to share a simultaneous orgasm.

If you make love with the same partner frequently, you'll soon develop your own favorite positions. Your choices will probably be dictated to some extent by the idiosyncrasies of your anatomies and how they fit, as well as which position best accommodates your sexual timing.

### Time Your Response Cycles

After some time making love together, you will learn approximately how long it takes for each of you to reach orgasm during your most typical lovemaking. Assuming it takes the woman longer than the man—and this is not always the case!—the man can stimulate the woman until she reaches the point where she is about as far away from climaxing as he will be when stimulation begins for him. It sounds like a lot of work, but some couples find the special intimacy of a simultaneous orgasm is well worth the effort.

# 8

# SECRETS OF THE ORIENT: TANTRIC AND TAOIST LOVEMAKING TECHNIQUES

Countless books, treatises, and essays about how to make love have been written by authors from all over the world. But two elaborately conceived advice tomes that date back to over two thousand years ago have had the most profound and enduring impact. The *Tao* of China and the *Kama Sutra* of India offer detailed and graphic information that is as relevant and enlightening—perhaps even more so—as any of today's writings. Perhaps this is so because tantric and Taoist sex instruction is an integral part of an entire philosophy of life. In addition, both books couch their advice in breathtakingly erotic language and images.

Tantric and Taoist followers view the sexual relationship as a sacred union that includes emotional bonds and is framed by a sense of spiritual oneness. The sex act is not a separate and distinct part of life; it flows from and expresses one's entire being. It is not a series of mechanical movements accomplished in order to reach orgasmic release as quickly as possible. Sexual satisfaction and health are part and parcel of a unified way of living that includes care of the body, mind, and soul, and the sense of self that comes from regular creative expression. Tantric and Taoist sex techniques not only make you a more skilled and happier lover, they can transform you entirely.

When you practice tantric and Taoist lovemaking, you are pleasure-oriented rather than goal-oriented, that is, unconcerned with "getting there," to orgasm. The experience becomes everything. Many of these lovemaking techniques are designed to extend lovemaking, to keep your arousal stoked at just below combustion point for as long as possible. This makes tantric and Taoist sex especially suitable for older men, who tend to need more time to become aroused and reach climax and can use the energy of sexual excitement to revitalize themselves. On the other hand, younger men also benefit; they acquire a greater degree of control over their sexuality than they ever believed possible.

Besides the tantric and Taoist sexual philosophies, another ancient Eastern lovemaking discipline known as *karezza* is thought to have originated in Persia (now Iran). *Karezza* basically involves lengthy periods of passive sexual intercourse—lying still for half an hour or more and allowing the male and female energies to build up and intermingle. Taoist lovemaking and, to a lesser extent, tantric lovemaking differ in that they encourage physical movement, which makes them more suitable to Westerners. *Karezza* also lacks the component of transforming sexual energy into a healing force. In short, *karezza* lovemaking is an effective antidote to goal-centered Western sex, but it does not offer as much pleasure or as many health benefits as do tantric and Taoist sex.

Tantric and Taoist sex practices require practice, discipline, and patience. But the rewards you reap are more than worth your efforts. And, in this case, the learning process is the greater part of your payoff in terms of fun and pleasure! Once you exchange the pressures of Western-style sexual striving for the ecstatic experience of Eastern-style lovemaking, you can enjoy, perhaps for the very first time, the most profound sexual passion and satisfaction.

The ancient love secrets you will master range from basic techniques that simply help you approach lovemaking from a new point of view to creating an ecstatic union of bodies and souls.

If you have been practicing Kegels, along with the Eastern exercises that tone and stimulate your sex organs and glands, your PC muscles should be strong, your libido turned on, and you should have gained control over your sexual energy. All these are prerequisites for Eastern-style lovemaking.

## Guidelines for Eastern Lovemaking

Before you follow any detailed instructions on tantric and Taoist lovemaking, read these general guidelines. Along with all the information you have received so far, these guidelines will further prepare you for the kind of passionate, exhilarating sex that enhances every other aspect of your life.

## MAKE LOVE AT THE RIGHT TIMES

Traditional Eastern disciplines teach that the best time for sex is the early morning, when your body is well rested. Of course, most of us are busy at that time, rushing to prepare children for school and ourselves for the workday. Nighttime is more convenient for those juggling the demands of work and family. But we are often tired or under emotional stress by the evening. So, it's a good idea to nap, rest, do a relaxation exercise or a visualization, or practice yoga in the evening before you draw on your sexual energy.

## USE THE BASIC EASTERN BREATH

Apply the breathing techniques you learned in chapter 4 to ensure that you deliver life-force energy deep into your lower abdomen, where it removes stress and revitalizes and sensitizes all your organs and glands, particularly those related to sex. You can also use this deep, regular nostril breathing either to awaken and accelerate your arousal or to calm you down whenever you get too close to climaxing.

## SYNCHRONIZE YOUR BREATHING

Breathing in unison puts your bodies and sexual energies in sync and increases your shared feelings of intimacy and union.

Petra and a lover "accidentally" stumbled onto this special and powerful sexual experience while making love one night on a deserted beach in the Caribbean. As they were locked together in a close embrace, their breathing spontaneously synchronized and they experienced the joy of true sexual union. It's been fifteen years since that magical night, but Petra has never forgotten it. "It was amazing, one of the most incredible experiences I've ever had," she says.

You don't have to wait for that magic to happen "accidentally." You can create that experience virtually any time you wish by following these simple instructions:

***LIE TOGETHER SPOON FASHION.*** If you are behind your partner, inhale through your belly as you visualize breathing in your partner's energy through his or her back.

***HOLD EACH OTHER CLOSELY.*** Position yourselves face to face, eyes shut, and deliberately breathe together for several minutes. Feel your bodies expand together with each inhalation and contract with each exhalation, as if you were one entity.

***BREATHE INTO EACH OTHER IN THE MIDST OF SEXUAL UNION.*** In the midst of intercourse, charge your excitement even higher by stopping all movement and pressing your faces together. Gaze into each other's eyes and bring your open mouths together. Exchange breaths, inhaling in your partner's exhalations and vice versa. This can be so arousing that you may feel compelled to kiss and dissolve into orgasm.

## Gaze Into Each Other's Eyes

Instead of closing your eyes while making love, look into each other's eyes and hold your gaze. This experience can be powerfully intimate; it can also provoke your vulnerability. Like virtually all tantric and Taoist lovemaking experiences, this level of intimacy is best shared with a partner whom you love and trust, because he or she will witness your innermost feelings as they express themselves through these "windows to the soul."

## Use the Nine Deep, One Shallow Pattern

This technique helps the man delay his orgasm and is very exciting for lovers. The man takes nine shallow strokes—so that only the head of the penis enters and stimulates the highly sensitive first third of the vagina—then one deep thrust—penetrating her completely. He never withdraws completely.

If his retreat is quicker than his slow penetration, the penis also contacts the clitoris, providing an added thrill.

### DON'T THRUST TOO VIGOROUSLY INTO THE VAGINA

Pounding away exhausts both of you and can hurt, even numb the vagina. Firm but gentle and varied thrusts are best.

### FIND THE SACRED SPOT

While mechanical-minded Westerners attempt to pin down the precise location of the G-spot, Easterners have always accepted that this sacred hot spot can shift position and even change size, depending on the woman's arousal level. He explores—as always, without the pressure of goals—and uses the woman's responses to guide him. Once he's found the center of her excitement, he massages the area with the come-hither gesture, until she ejaculates a clear, sweet-smelling liquid.

### STIMULATE YOUR IMAGINATION BEFOREHAND

Tuning into your partner one to two days before lovemaking can help you build a higher arousal level. If there are any issues or feelings of anger or anxiety, work on them by feeding yourself positive suggestions and viewing positive visualizations, such as those you learned in chapter 5, on the movie screen of your mind. Always make love in an atmosphere of calm.

### SET THE SCENE FOR ROMANCE

Your lovemaking should take place in a romantic, relaxed atmosphere, with dim lighting or candlelight, loose, silken-textured clothing, perfumes and other sweet scents, and soft, sensual music.

### DON'T MAKE LOVE ON A FULL BLADDER

Urinate before lovemaking, then wait at least twenty minutes so that the organs involved get a brief rest period. Also, never make love on a full stomach. Sex on a full belly is not good for your digestion or your love life.

### Don't Make Love When Drunk on Alcohol or High on Drugs

When you're drunk or high, you're out of control. You may think you need to be inebriated in order to get past your fears and other blocks about sex. But Taoist and tantric lovemaking are about retaining a certain degree of control within the context of true sexual freedom. One or two drinks may help you shed the tensions of the day, but drunkenness can actually become harmful to your health when you are practicing tantric and Taoist lovemaking.

### Don't Engage in Hard Physical Work Before or After Sex

Sexual activity draws on your energy, as does hard physical labor. Always make sure you are rested before making love and that you rest afterward.

### Don't Bathe or Shower Immediately After Sex

Water draws off much of the electrical charge you have built up together. (Yes! You may not see it but many holistic healers affirm that lovemaking does build up an electric charge that radiates from the partners.) Wait until you have relaxed and your body has absorbed this energy.

### Minimize the Use of Sex Toys Such as Vibrators and Dildos

The danger in sex toys is that you can become overly reliant on artificial sex aids. It is always better to increase your capacity for sexual pleasure through a healthy and strengthening diet, the right exercise program, and relaxation and visualization techniques.

### If Sex Has Become Routine, Take a Break

Stop making love for a while. When you resume, give your lovemaking a special boost by trying out either the Taoist or tantric union, both of which are described below.

## SHARING A VALLEY ORGASM

This is where you reap all the benefits of all your study and practice thus far. The Valley Orgasm brings together every technique you learned in chapters 4 through 7 so you can enjoy the most powerful sexual experience possible. In fact, in order to have a Valley Orgasm, it is also essential that you follow the nutritional advice in chapters 1 through 3 and practice the exercises and techniques in chapter 4, in order to prepare your body to handle the intense sensations of the Valley Orgasm and the in-flow of life-force energy it creates. You will also call on the visualization powers you developed by practicing the techniques described in chapter 5 so that you can gather and direct your aroused energy to create a unified energy circuit that joins you and your lover. All this will help you transform ordinary, perfunctory sex into an experience of unparalleled bliss.

The following are step-by-step instructions on how to have Valley Orgasms:

1. Begin active intercourse, alternating nine shallow thrusts with one deep thrust.

2. As each of you or both of you approach orgasm, stop movement. The man should withdraw his penis, but never completely, then both of you practice the Taoist Energy Transformation in order to draw the aroused energy you've cultivated up each of your spines.

Inhale deeply and visualize pulling your aroused energy up from your genitals through your spine. (Eventually, you will draw it up to your brain.)

4. Make a loud sigh or moan as your exhale, and the energy will continue peaking and moving upward on its own.

Hold each other closely as you exhale. Then relax and synchronize your breathing.

5. Each time both your arousal levels drop by half, begin active intercourse again to rebuild your store of energy.

6. Each time either or both of you is about to come, stop moving and direct that energy upward.

7. Repeat this process several times, each time gathering more and more energy and bringing it further and further up your spines.

8. Call on your visualization powers to see that energy as a stream of light, as you both continue to inhale, exhale, and move that aroused energy upward. You will eventually create a circle of energy that either travels through your bodies or around them.
9. Once the energy has reached both your brains, share an orgasmic tongue press, in which you press your tongues together to complete the energy circuit that initiated with genital contact.

To keep the energy pumping, the woman should rhythmically contract and relax her vaginal, PC, and anal muscles, while the man contracts and relaxes his PC and anal muscles. Pump as your tongues are pressed together for as long as you can, until the energy makes a complete circuit of both your bodies.

Each time you allow sexual desire to rebuild and then redirect it upward, the sensation of this higher orgasm becomes increasingly intense and pleasurable. It is radically different from "lower" or "outward," genital orgasms in that you feel it in every part of your body, and you gain, rather than lose, vital energy.

Again, ejaculation and orgasm are two separate and distinct experiences. Your orgasm can last as long as you desire and travel as high as you direct it. Once you've ejaculated, though, your orgasm is gone. You can avoid ejaculating altogether or experience a few Valley Orgasms and then conclude with a "regular," outward-discharging orgasm.

When you are ready to share a Valley Orgasm with an equally prepared and willing partner, a wonderful new world opens up to you. But never engage in this type of lovemaking with someone who doesn't know these techniques; you could actually drain energy from that person and do him or her harm.

It may be especially hard to convince a male partner to hold back his ejaculation, and many men require a great deal of solo practice. The woman can help by serving as a positive guide and coach. Here are some other methods a man can use to delay ejaculation.

## FURTHER TIPS FOR DELAYING EJACULATION

### *Push Down*

This temporary "emergency" measure is similar to the Kegel bear-down and can be used by men and women. Push down as if you were having a bowel movement—but not too forcefully! It should feel as if your genitals are bulging slightly, and you will naturally hold your breath. Don't make a regular practice of this technique, as doing it too frequently or too vigorously could weaken your muscles.

### *Testicle Ring*

Make a ring with your thumb and forefinger as you grasp the skin between the testicles and the body and pull downward.

### *Cold Water Skinny Dip*

This one takes a bit of courage. Have a bowl of cold water by the bed so that the man can immerse his penis for an instant cool down.

### *Count Slowly*

This technique seems to have spread through the world; just about every man knows it. As your orgasm threatens to overtake you, cool off by counting from 1 to 100, slowly.

## EASTERN LOVE RITUAL

This beautifully orchestrated, ritualistic union allows you to draw on all your new skills, including your ability to transform fantasy into reality and to enjoy sexual role playing. It is one of the most thrilling erotic adventures you'll ever undertake. Some of its aspects may strike you as hokey, even ridiculous—impossible to do without collapsing in giggles. If so, either giggle your way through or eliminate those elements of the Eastern Love Ritual and enjoy the rest.

The deliberateness, slow pace, role playing, and respect paid to the woman in this love ritual are effective antidotes to our usual Western style of rushed, straining sex. This experience not only promotes greater awareness and sensitivity to your body's sensations; it enhances health and promotes feelings of love, devotion, and tenderness between the partners.

Again, it's hard to imagine such an intimate experience with anyone other than someone you love and trust.

## THE EASTERN LOVE RITUAL: STEP BY STEP

First, choose the ideal time for you and your lover to share this experience. Create a romantic setting where this union will take place. The lighting should be dim but not totally dark. You can use a corner of your bedroom or part of another room and transform it into a bower of love by hanging luxurious fabrics, putting up other wall decorations, and placing vases full of fragrant flowers and scented candles in attractive holders all around. If you use a lamp, try to find a violet shade, a violet light bulb, or drape the lamp with violet fabric—safely! (Remember, violet energizes and harmonizes the female sex organs and glands.)

Cover the bed, floor, or couch—which should be comfortable yet firm—with a special spread.

Arrange a tray with a bowl of bite-size pieces of fruit, a pitcher of pure water and two glasses, a bottle of your favorite liqueur and two liqueur glasses, and a dish containing your favorite sweet treats, such as chocolates, marzipan, or some other especially delicious candy, cookies, or cake.

Bathe thoroughly, not only for obvious esthetic and hygienic reasons, but so the bioelectrical currents of your bodies can flow freely between you. Anoint yourselves with your favorite natural perfume oils and then dress.

The man enters the place of love and lights the candles, then does a yoga or Taoist breathing exercise to calm his body and center his mind. Between inhalations and exhalations, he holds his breath and simultaneously contracts the muscles of his anus. As he does this, he anticipates the union that is to take place as one that will be shared by a god and a goddess.

He invites his partner in, and she sits by his side, in front of the table-altar holding the tray of food and drink. The man fills the liqueur glasses and passes one to the woman. They lift their glasses in unison and take a sip. Each partner then takes a small piece of fruit from the plate and they eat. They take another sip of liqueur, then eat a piece of candy or cake.

At this point, do any of the following: One or both of you—taking turns—can dance for the other, either robed or disrobed. Gaze into your partner's eyes as you move to your favorite music. Undulate your torso, feel your abdomen and pelvis relax, open, and fill with life-giving energy. You can also dance together—apart or in a close embrace. Mirror each other's movements, beginning with one mirroring the other, then switch and continue until it's impossible to detect who is the initiator and who is the follower.

Have fun, play, and remember to keep breathing deeply and evenly into your belly. Allow any sounds to come out: sighs, growls, pants, groans, giggles. Avoid words, as they tend to take you out of your body and into your "head." End the dancing with a deep, body-to-body hug in which each of you nestles closely into each other's body. Then step back a bit and gaze into each other's eyes.

Leave the table and go to the bed, couch, or floor. The woman disrobes, except perhaps for jewelry, and sits upright on the edge of the bed. The man stands before her.

The violet lamp is lit and angled so that its light falls on the woman's nude pelvis. The man gazes on her with admiration and awe, as if pondering the mystery of creation and the secret of being. He must see his partner as a treasure-house of beauty, the source of creation. If he cannot see her in this way, do not go any further.

Lie down together and take turns lightly stroking each other's body. Use a feather or featherlike strokes of the fingertips. The woman can use her hair to brush up and down the length of the man's body and then across it. Breathe slowly and deeply. Imagine energy flowing out your fingertips, the feather, or your hair, and into your partner's body.

A good alternative is to massage each other, using a scented vegetable oil. Follow the massage instructions given in chapter 6. You can finish the massage with both of you rolling around, sliding and rubbing your oiled bodies together.

The woman then reclines on her back while the man lies on his left side, facing her. The woman raises both her legs by bending her knees and pulling them upward toward her chest. The man then swings the upper part of his body away from hers and brings his penis in close contact with her vagina. She then lowers her legs, and he places his right leg between her legs. The maneuver brings the sex organs of the partners in close contact. You can stay like this as long as your wish.

The man gently parts the labia and partially inserts his penis—not deeply.

At this point, follow either of the next steps to complete the Eastern Love Ritual:

To make this a tantric union, both partners lie completely motionless and relaxed for a period of a half hour as they visualize the flow of energy between them, the strongest being at the point of genital contact. Gradually, each partner will become aware of a rising tide of pleasure that keeps growing in intensity, as more and more energy builds and courses through the sex organs and up the spine. Near the end of the half hour, the sensation will peak, resulting in an involuntary orgasm that will involve contractions of the entire body.

After this simultaneous orgasm, sexual tension naturally recedes, and both partners are left with an ineffable sense of wholeness, peace, and unity.

If the man feels he is about to ejaculate during this union, he can prevent it by holding his breath, at the same time turning his tongue backward as far as he can against the roof of his mouth and contracting his anal muscles. Or he can use any of the other ejaculation prevention techniques given above and in previous chapters.

If the man does ejaculate, the union ends, because the energy has been dispersed through that outward orgasm and is no longer available to move up into both partners' bodies. Try again another evening.

This tantric union can go on for two or three hours, and ends either by the man's withdrawal or when both partners naturally fall asleep.

To make this a Taoist union, follow the instructions given above on how to have Valley Orgasms.

The Eastern Love Union is not a substitute for "regular" lovemaking, but it's a wonderful ritual to practice once a month or so to keep your relationship exciting and vibrant.

# 9

# FANTASIES, GAMES, AND EROTICA

All the information you've read so far will help you enjoy your body in new, wonderfully sensuous ways. If you've started practicing the various exercises and applying the many tips you've learned, you should have already experienced a noticeable boost in your love life. The Eastern Love Ritual that concludes the previous chapter draws on the most potent sex charger of all—your imagination. Your imagination's ability to galvanize your sexual desire and enhance your lovemaking pleasures is virtually unlimited. Sexual fantasies, games, and other erotica—the subject of this chapter—are the icing on your love cake, powerful turn-ons that work on your mind.

You learned in previous chapters to use your imagination to create images that enhance your sexuality. Here, you will read about sharing fantasies, role playing, and indulging in erotic games. Sharing fantasies and role playing with your partner are among the most effective ways to heat up your love life together and add the spice of variety to a long-term relationship.

## SEXUAL FANTASY

Sexual fantasies can range from a brief glimpse into someone's eyes accompanied by the momentary question about what that person would be like in bed to elaborately planned and staged romantic scenarios like the Eastern Love Ritual. Fantasies typically involve a steamy setting, playing sexually provocative characters, acting out a lengthy seduction, and slow, lingering lovemaking—

and any other element that stirs your passion. Some people even have favorite fantasies, like scenes from a movie, that they rewind and play over and over again.

A fantasy that involves role playing can transform a bland, routine encounter into sizzling, unforgettable lovemaking. In fact, any couple that has been together for a long time will invariably benefit from some form of sexual fantasy and role playing. If your sex life has become predictable and humdrum, your first strategy should be to check your fantasy life together, then use the power of your imaginations to lift you out of that rut. Do you even have a fantasy life together?

Aaron and his fiancée were fighting all the time and not getting along in bed at all. "We were lying to each other," Aaron recalls. "We were pretending to each other that we were sexually satisfied, but we weren't. I thought she was no longer attracted to me, and she thought I wasn't attracted to her.

"One day we went for a drive and we somehow began to trade sexual fantasies. I was pleasantly surprised to realize that she still wanted me and that her fantasy about what she wanted me to do to her actually turned me on. I shared with her that I'd been dying to come all over her breasts. We became so excited that we couldn't wait to get home and tear off each other's clothes."

If you are having trouble coming up with your own original fantasies, draw your inspiration from erotic literature, tapes, and films—especially if you and your partner read and watch them together. Erotica can also help you discover what really turns you on.

## Erotic Books and Videotapes

It wasn't so long ago that "pornographic" films were roughly made black-and-white affairs viewed in secret by men only in dark, smoky backrooms. Today's women are freer about their sexuality, which has led to a boom in the newest sector of the erotic video business—movies designed primarily to arouse women. The same is true of erotic literature; more and more books are written with women and couples in mind, for entertainment and sex instruction purposes alike.

While many men and women are excited by the same fantasies and images, women tend to prefer more romantic themes and a good story line. "If a man likes it, it's porn," says Ivan, a thirty-one-year-old businessman. "For a woman it's erotica."

Erotica crosses the line and becomes offensive and dangerous pornography when the sexually explicit and arousing material involves sex acts with children or violence to a sex partner.

The Resource Guide includes lists of the most popular erotic books.

## TOP SEXUAL FANTASIES

The following are fantasies experts say are the most common, along with some examples of people's individual variations on these popular themes. Use them as they are, or as a springboard to create your own original scenarios.

### MAKING LOVE WITH SOMEONE NEW

"I believe in reincarnation," says Sharon, "and in a former life I'm sure I was a prostitute with multiple sex partners. Now my greatest fantasy is lying in bed, with men lined up from my bedroom to several blocks away, and I just say, 'Next! Next!' That's it!"

### MAKING LOVE WITH A FORBIDDEN PARTNER—SOMEONE FROM ANOTHER RACE OR CLASS, A FRIEND'S SPOUSE

Janis and her best friend's ex, Peter, have always felt a subtle sexual attraction to each other, but Janis was afraid of hurting her friend. Janis's favorite fantasy involves being trapped with Peter all night long in a stalled elevator. Since the elevator is in an office building, and it's after working hours, they both realize no one will come to free them until morning. The elevator is large and carpeted, and Janis just happens to have food and water with her, left over from lunch. So neither of them is too afraid. As the hours pass, though, the temperature rises, and the heat finally forces them to strip naked. They glance at each other's nude, glistening bodies, then quickly look away. Neither says a word, but their pulses quicken. Janis is sure Peter can hear her heart thudding. A few moments tick by before Peter finally grabs Janis in a rough, passionate embrace, and they melt together in a deep kiss. They slide down to the floor and make wild, sweaty love all night long, until they are "rescued" in the early morning.

### Making Love with Two or More Other People—A Male Favorite

Robert's fantasy begins with a king-size bed covered by a rubber sheet, over which he pours scented massage oil. Two gorgeous women make love to each other on the bed while he watches. "They're doing this for me," he explains. "They're enjoying each other, but they keep looking over at me to see my reaction and smiling seductively. As I watch, I prepare myself. Then, they request my presence—no, *demand* my presence. They massage me from head to toe with their entire bodies. Finally, we indulge in extended foreplay with lots of teasing, and finish with an explosive, three-way climax."

### Making Love in an Exotic, Faraway Locale—A Moonlit Beach, a Penthouse Balcony, in a Private Jet Plane

Jason's ultimate fantasy is to be moored on a fabulous yacht with all the amenities, about 150 miles out at sea, off the shores of an exotic Caribbean island. He and his three male friends and four voluptuous women can barely glimpse land. "It's about six p.m., and the sun is just beginning its descent in the West," says Jason. "We're fishing, but we occasionally jump into the sea to refresh ourselves and sip glasses of champagne in which grapes and almonds are floating. The sounds of soft reggae and R and B music float in the gentle breeze."

As darkness falls and the stars light up the sky, each of the four couples wanders away to find a romantic, secluded spot to make passionate love all night.

### Making Love with a Stranger, on the Spur of the Moment—On a Train or Plane

Carl travels a good deal for his business. His fantasy begins on a train, as he exchanges glances with a gorgeous woman wearing a beautifully fitted, ultra-chic business suit. The looks grow bolder and longer as time passes. "Finally, the woman gets up from her seat, looks at me, then looks meaningfully in the direction of the bathroom," Carl says. "I understand that I am to follow her there. We make hurried, frantic, incredibly hot love standing up. Then we straighten our clothes and tidy our hair, go back to our respective seats, and behave as if nothing had happened."

### Making Love Under Force

You can sleep with anyone you want and you don't have to feel guilty! After all, you were forced. "I can think of nothing more wonderful than being blindfolded and confined to a bed," giggles Joyce. "Eight people take turns doing me at the same time—in various combinations. I can't do anything to stop them. After a while, I don't want to!"

### Making Love in Forbidden Spots Where You Could Easily Be Discovered—Behind a Bush in a Public Park, in a Public Washroom, a Swimming Pool, in the Sea

Ellen was traveling in Italy when she came upon a lush, expansive park in Rome. All she could think about was how exciting it would be to duck under a bush or behind a tree with a darkly handsome Roman and make deliciously furtive love. "People stroll past us," she says, elaborating on her fantasy. "But they're completely unaware of what is going on only a few yards away."

### Making Love with Someone of the Same Sex

Lynne has never made love with another woman. "But one of my favorite fantasies is to make love with my mirror image—the brunette counterpart to my own blond beauty," she says. "It would be like being myself and my dopplegänger at the same time—doubling my pleasure."

### Watching Your Partner Make Love to Someone Else

Although he would never accept his fantasy in real life, Jim has always wanted to watch his girlfriend, Beth, making love. "The only way I could see *every* move she makes and *every* expression of her passion is if she were making love to another man—an extremely virile-looking body builder type," Jason explains. "Of course, Beth would be doing this only to please me. Her mind would be constantly on my excitement, and even during the heights of her passion, her eyes would never leave mine."

### Making Love with a Celebrity

Ever since Jane saw a sixties film adaptation of Faulkner's *Sanctuary*, about a privileged Southern belle who is imprisoned by a French brothel keeper and eventually becomes his willing love slave, she began fantasizing about its star, the late sexy French film actor and singer Yves Montand. "For decades now—even after Montand became a gray-haired senior citizen—my favorite sexual fantasy has been to imagine myself playing out the exact same scenario—enslaved by lust to Yves Montand."

### Spanking Each Other Lightly for Some Imaginary Misdeed or Another

Donna and her boyfriend enjoy this harmless punishment fantasy. Whenever she is in the mood, she greets him at the door wearing a girlishly provocative outfit. "I've been a bad girl!" she'll announce with a little smile. He asks her in a mock-stern tone to describe her transgression. She does and her boyfriend replies that her punishment will be a spanking, which, of course, inevitably leads to a night of lovemaking.

### Dress Up as Characters You Find Sexy

You can play spy-seductress and victim or schoolgirl and the principal, or prostitute and John. That last one is especially fun in public. Any roles you find appealing will do. Then drive each other crazy with desire. Take your time teasing and tempting.

Kevin and his girlfriend like to play police and thief. He breaks and enters, and just as he's filling his bag with jewelry and other valuables, he feels her gun stuck in his back.

"She tells me to put my hands behind my back and she handcuffs me," Kevin explains. "I realize from the sound of her voice that she's a woman. She tells me, 'You could get twenty years for this.'

"'Isn't there anything else we can do?' I beg, trying to broker a deal.

"'I'm a detective and I make good money,' she answers, 'but we can make another kind of deal.'

"She pushes me onto the couch on my back. 'Let's have a good look at you,' she says, as she rips off my ski mask and tears my shirt open, then undoes the fly on my pants.

"She performs oral sex on me, then straddles my body and rides me like a bucking bronco."

### Switch Roles

If the woman pretends to be the man and the man pretends to be the woman, you can enjoy a funny and erotic seduction fantasy. The woman gets to be aggressive, and the man gets to be passive. "I was the man and I had to convince him to give me some," says Janis, laughing at the memory. "It was so much fun and so hot, because I had the opportunity to go into a male psyche. It was very liberating and contradictory, because I'm usually in the opposite position—the one being persuaded. This time, I had to pull all these schemes out of my head to get him to give in. I lied to him, made promises, told him anything—anything he wanted to hear—so he would give me some."

## *Creating Your Own Fantasies*

Acting out exciting sexual fantasies that you created yourself is even more fun and much easier than you may believe. Studies suggest that today, more than ever, men and women are having similar fantasies, possibly because modern women are freer about their sexuality and enjoy being sexual, explicit, and even aggressive in bed. If you and your partner tend to respond to the same imaginative turn-ons, the process of coscripting and acting out your own fantasy—tailor-made for the two of you—could be your most exciting sexual adventure yet.

Lisa was training to be a chef at a famous culinary institute, so most of her sex fantasies were food-related—a common association. One evening she invited her boyfriend Eric over for dinner. He rang the bell, and Lisa answered the door as if she was the maitre d' and her home was an upscale restaurant. She escorted him to his table and handed him the menu she'd written up in neat, attractive calligraphy.

"There were three courses," Eric recalls. "She'd cooked everything from scratch. That was a big turn-on, to know she'd spent the entire day shopping for food and cooking, just to present it all to me.

"The first two courses were served in the living room. Dessert was served in the bedroom . . . on her abdomen. It was cheesecake with lots of cherries and cherry sauce. No one ever since has been as deep and open a lover. With her, it was okay to say, 'I want to cover your breasts with chocolate sauce.'

"Even if I said that to a woman today, over fifteen years later, we probably wouldn't get around to actually doing it. Too busy these days."

## Games to Heat Up Your Love Life

Playing games together can restore your youthful sense of fun, creativity, and freedom. Too often we lose those qualities as we grow older and take on the responsibilities of adults. But sex does not have to be serious business all the time. Laughter belongs in the bedroom, along with sighs and moans of pleasure, and a fun-filled sexual experience can be wonderfully liberating.

Arlene and Keith, a couple who lived together in New York City, hit upon their favorite game after visiting Arlene's brother in the suburbs and observing her two nieces playing hide and seek. They decided to play the game in their loft apartment—in the nude. Arlene hid first, and Keith had to find her, then chase her

Write some scenarios together and some separately. Then get together and act them out.

When Steve was a university student, he and his girlfriend had one class together. "It was the healthiest sexual relationship of my life," he says. "We'd write each other notes describing our fantasies and what we wanted to do to each other. It was much easier than describing them face to face. We'd exchange notes during our class. Then, after classes finished, we'd go to her place and act them out. One day we'd act out my fantasy, the next day hers."

You can exchange written descriptions of your fantasies like Steve and his girlfriend. Or, you can describe several fantasies, each on separate pieces of paper. Fold the papers, put them in a bowl, then take turns closing your eyes and picking out a paper. Then act that fantasy out.

back to home base. Soon, they were shrieking with excitement, and after only one round, they wound up in bed and enjoyed their best sex in over a year.

Hide and seek in the nude or any of the following sex games will definitely restore a sense of lightheartedness and excitement to your love life:

- Throw a love banquet. This game is a particularly effective way to persuade a squeamish partner to give oral sex. Take a shower together first, then smear your favorite treats all over each other. Take turns feasting on each other's mouth-watering bodies. Try spreading your love feast on less explored erogenous zones, so you and your lover can lick, nibble, suck, and chew new places. Use your hands to stroke and caress your lover while your mouth, tongue, and lips nibble away. This is not only great fun; it is instructive. You can use the same sensuous moves on your lover any time, not just when you're using food. Make sure to go gently around the sensitive sex organs—the vulva and clitoris, and the penis and testicles. Don't worry about calories—pile on the whipped cream, chocolate sauce, and peanut butter. You're sure to work it off.

Melanie's husband gave her a creative Valentine's Day gift. He brought home a triple chocolate cake from their favorite bakery, and they spent a delirious evening eating the scrumptious dessert off each other's bodies.

• Warm weather presents many opportunities for *al fresco* game playing, followed by lovemaking. Secluded parks, camping, and hiking trips, mountain climbing—sex on a mountain peak—the top of the world! All these scenarios make for amorous outdoor adventure. You can also turn your love feast into an outdoor picnic, especially on a warm, starlit night. Just make sure your privacy is assured.

• Number different areas of each other's bodies—the back of the neck, the inside of the thigh, armpits, toes. Try to pinpoint new "hot spots." Then write the numbers on separate scraps of paper and throw them into a hat or bowl. Take turns picking numbers and having the other partner kiss and lick each numbered spot for a while.

• Play the game Twister (where you have to assume some interesting positions) in the nude.

• Play a rousing game of that old standard, strip poker or strip monopoly. The game ends when someone is completely nude. That's also when lovemaking begins.

• Feather tickle each other—all over, or on those numbered spots. Do it nice and slow.

• Discover the erotic delights of body painting. The gentle, featherlike sensations of the paint brush moving over your body increases your sensual awareness and makes for a sexually exciting and creatively fulfilling experience. If you really get into this, experiment with air brushes, tiny paint brushes, and painting through various nets and fabrics to produce a variety of beautiful designs and styles.

• Apply Emotion Lotion. Apply this special love lotion to your lover's body, then gently blow on his/her skin for a warm tingling sensation. Switch places.

• Initiate royalty nights. Take turns playing king or queen while the other acts as humble love servant—serving a meal, giving a massage, drawing a scented bath. Wind up by fulfilling his or her every sexual whim. Or you can gamble for "slave nights." Winner gets the slave. You can even include a little light bondage—excellent for provoking harmless fantasies of dominance and surrender.

• Watch erotic videos and follow the actors' lead, right along with them. Be sure to point out what turns *you* on. You can also reenact your favorite movie sex scene or some time when the two of you were together that was especially sexy.

• Make your own private erotic tapes.

• Have a watermelon fight in the nude, or choose any other juicy, slippery, tasty food as your weapon.

• Give him a nice, long lap dance. You do everything, while he just holds onto the chair for the ride of his life. If necessary, tie him there. All he is allowed to do is kiss back.

• Do a striptease for him, but don't take it all off—at least not too quickly. Undress slowly and tantalizingly and do it to your favorite hot music.

• Decide that you're only going to touch each other for an hour. No kissing, no genital stimulation. It's amazing how erotic this is. Touch everywhere. Remember, the entire body is your erotic playground. Feel as if you are touching each other for the very first time.

• Try sucking on an ice cube, then giving your partner oral sex. Some women enjoy oral sex with ice cubes inserted in their vaginas.

## WHEN FANTASIES AND GAMES ARE GOOD FOR YOU AND WHEN THEY'RE NOT

Playing games and spinning out fantasies as a prelude to or part of lovemaking enhances the erotic mood and helps you forget your usual worries, tensions, and inhibitions. It is perfectly safe and harmless. However, some of us have difficulty in accepting our true sexual desires and fantasies.

Do not confuse the sexual fantasies that spontaneously come to mind with your actual sexual wishes. In fact, few of us would want to see our fantasies play out in real life. For example, fantasizing about being forced to have sex does not mean you want to be raped in real life.

You might feel guilty because you fantasize about sexual acts you consider wrong or immoral, such as committing adultery or engaging in a homosexual or sadomasochistic encounter.

Religious teachings or parental messages may have instilled in you the notion that sex is "dirty."

You might think that your adultery fantasy means you've sinned in thought, even though you haven't committed the actual deed.

You could also fear that if you *really* let your imagination go, you will become totally corrupted and go off the sexual deep end.

None of these fears and worries are valid unless your fantasies are disrupting your relationship. Try to view them as little vacations from reality and enjoy these breaks. Daydreams that involve unusual sexual scenarios or many or strange bed partners are perfectly normal and safe because they *are* fantasies.

Keep in mind at all times that fantasy is not reality. There's no need for guilt or regrets because nothing *actually* happens!

There are warning signs, though, that let you know when your fantasy is not healthy.

### If You Are Dependent on a Well-worn Fantasy

If you *always* need to replay your fantasy to get you going, and you cannot become sexually aroused or reach orgasm without replaying this fantasy every time you have sex, you do have a problem.

Overreliance on fantasy to become sexually excited keeps you "in your head" and isolates your erotic life from the rest of your life experience. Sexual excitement mainly results from the very real physical sensations of aroused energy building in the sex organs and moving throughout your body.

If your mind fixates on air-brushed media images of male and female sexual perfection—often created by artificial enhancements such as implants, liposuction, and other "miracles" of modern cosmetic surgery, as well as modern photo-enhancement techniques—you move even further away from the profound and rejuvenating *real* experience of true sexual feelings. And if your partner or you don't measure up to these unreal standards of beauty, you can become dissatisfied with your sex life together.

The Eastern Love Ritual and other Eastern sex exercises are effective antidotes to overreliance on fantasy. If your fantasies are too hard to resist, Taoist experts recommend that you immerse yourself in them completely, even act them out during sex (that is, if they are not dangerous), until you naturally purge yourself of their hold on you. Since fantasies rarely live up to expectations once they're acted out in real life, especially repeatedly, they eventually lose their attraction.

### If Your Fantasies Always Contain Themes of Violence

Sexual fantasies can sometimes get a bit violent and bizarre. But if *all* your fantasies have a violent theme, you should be worried. If this is your case, it is essential that you seek professional counseling to help you better understand those fantasies and replace them with healthier themes.

## The Erotic Internet

The Internet is a private and relatively safe way to explore sexual fantasies and share experiences through on-line sex discussion groups. In the privacy of your own home, you can be as open as you desire in sharing your fantasies, preferences, or seeking information from others. Couples whose computers are linked to video camera images also enjoy sharing their digital images with other couples.

There are certain safety issues linked to these types of friendships. You never *really* know who is behind the image or words on your computer screen. Never give out your telephone number or address or agree to meet a new Internet friend anywhere other than a well-trafficked public location. These few guidelines will ensure that you do not place yourself in any danger.

## Sex Toys

Sex toys include vibrators, dildos, feathers, various forms of restraints, ben wa balls (small steel balls that are inserted into the vagina that you can also use to perform the Taoist vaginal strengthening exercises described in chapter 4), cock rings, even whips, paddles, costumes, and nipple clamps, and the accoutrements of S & M. Any object used to arouse a partner and/or prolong and intensify lovemaking falls into the category of sex toys. More and more people are using sex toys these days, because it's no longer necessary to buy them in person. The many mail-order businesses that specialize in sex toys means that you don't have to pay an embarrassing visit to a store you might consider sleazy. These items can even be ordered off the Internet. In addition, many of these toys and erotica are increasingly geared to appeal to women.

Many women have learned about their own sexuality and have had their first orgasms with a vibrator, and many continue to find it easier to orgasm with a vibrator. It's very common for couples to experiment with vibrators and other sex toys.

Keep in mind, though, that overreliance on mechanical devices can actually impede your true sexual happiness.

### *Keeping It Real with a Vibrator*

If you do use a vibrator or other sex toys, here are some pointers to help you avoid turning sex into a purely mechanical experience:

- Be sure to caress and kiss each other to maintain your emotional bond.
- Try different types of toys to see which experience suits the both of you.
- Don't forget to use lubrication, which makes the experience more comfortable and lifelike.
- Don't go straight for the genitals. Begin by using the device as a massage tool.
- Combine intercourse with the vibrator on her clitoris or his perineum.

## Reluctant Partners

Your partner or even you may be reluctant to share fantasies, role play, experiment with sex toys, or experience erotica. For example, you may be reluctant to share your fantasies because you fear shocking or offending your partner. You could even be afraid of boring or disappointing your partner with a pedestrian fantasy that involves nothing more than a romantic candlelit dinner, wine, a blindfolded violin trio, a massage, and slow, lingering caresses.

Try not to let those negative thoughts inhibit you and keep you from playing games and enjoying fantasies that can widen your sexual horizons. Fantasies and games allow you to explore new territory that you might otherwise consider taboo. Since role playing is usually involved, you are not being your "ordinary," everyday self. You're like an actor who's playing "a character," which is a great way to give yourself permission to break free of your usual sexual restrictions.

What do you do if your partner doesn't want to act out fantasies, play erotic games, or share erotica with you?

- If your partner is reluctant to play games and enjoy fantasies with you, create a special game or fantasy just for him or her. This can make your partner feel freer and perhaps even go on to create his or her own fantasy or game.
- Be sensitive to your lover and gauge how comfortable he or she would be with your particular fantasy. The main consideration at all times should be your partner's feelings.
- Don't pressure him or her. A good first step is to watch an erotic video by yourself, making sure to leave the door open so that he or she can wander into the room.
- If your partner does agree, for instance, to watch an erotic video or read erotic literature with you, choose something he or she would like or ask your partner to make the choice for both of you. You can also prescreen a few selections and choose the one you both would enjoy best.
- Make sure you do not make any negative comparisons between your lover and an actor, and don't make a big deal about how great someone's body is. Many women are threatened by the often unrealistic perfection of the actresses in erotic videos. Men are usually less affected than women, but they can also be threatened by the actors' penis sizes.
- Assure your partner that if, at any time, he or she feels uncomfortable, you will turn off the video or stop reading aloud.

# 10

# NATURAL APHRODISIACS

The human quest for a magic elixir that will turn men into unstoppable satyrs and women into insatiable vixens is at least as old as the search for the fountain of youth and the formula that transforms lead into gold. Aphrodisiacs—substances that, when ingested or applied to the skin, increase sexual desire—have inspired countless myths and old wives tales through the ages.

Truth and fiction mingle freely when it comes to the claims made for exotic concoctions that are quaffed by millions in the hopes of transforming their sex lives. The Caribbean man, for instance, favors brews of the seaweed Irish moss and linseed and concoctions of cow and goat parts and other exotic nutrients. These aphrodisiacs bear colorfully descriptive names like "magnum force" and "strong back."

In China, men dine on sea slugs, whose reputation for enhancing potency comes from their tendency to swell up when touched. Other delicacies reputed to enhance sexual performance include beheaded partridge, hippopotamus snout, and any phallic-shaped food substance that is dipped in oil, pepper, and nettle seeds. The *Kama Sutra* claims that eating "many eggs fried in butter, then immersed in honey, will make the member hard for the whole night."

Other substances alleged to have aphrodisiac powers by various peoples during various periods in recorded history include oysters, powdered rhino horn, cocaine, marijuana, alcohol, asparagus, pomegranates, and figs.

Between the overblown fantasies of believers and the blanket dismissals of disbelievers is the reality that certain foods, supplements, and herbs are, in fact, scientifically proven to enhance sex drive, endurance, and pleasure. Since low libido is most often due to nutritional deficiencies, the so-called aphrodisiacs designed to be taken over the long term to support the health and function of the sex organs and glands are really tonics. True aphrodisiacs are taken half an hour to an hour before having sex. Their purpose is to stimulate the libido for the short term. But there are no elixirs that can work sexual miracles, and some substances that claim to be aphrodisiacs are actually quite dangerous.

The truth is, if you're interested in revving up your libido, you can forget about specific pills and potions if you're not healthy. If you're in relatively good shape—eating right, exercising, and taking supplements and herbs that strengthen the sex organs and glands and the body overall, you shouldn't need an aphrodisiac—especially if you've been following the recommendations given in part 1 of this book. You should be so charged with natural sexual energy that you don't need any extra help!

However, there are times in the lives of even the most fit and vibrant person when the demands of work and family and other stresses slow him or her down. If you find yourself in a temporary energy and libido slump, certain natural aphrodisiacs can give you the lift you need.

Of course, if low or fluctuating hormone levels are your problem, taking hormone supplements or applying ProGest cream will raise and balance your hormone levels and produce an aphrodisiaclike effect. This is particularly true in the case of menopausal women who frequently discover that hormone replacement therapy (HRT) restores their sex drive. For instance, small doses of testosterone, the male sex hormone present in both sexes, is also used by some doctors to restore sexual desire in older men and women. Chapter 12 discusses the pros and cons of HRT more thoroughly, as well as your natural alternative options.

On the other hand, if you suffer from nutritional deficiencies and a weakened urogenital system, many tonic and aphrodisiac foods, supplements, and herbs—and even hormone therapy—will work first to strengthen and tone you. You won't notice any change in sexual desire, performance, or satisfaction until these deficiencies are made up. Once you have done so, you can experiment with the natural libido-boosting substances described in this chapter.

## Seduction and Scents

Over the centuries and in all cultures, we human beings have known almost instinctively to use scent on our bodies and clothing in order to increase our sexual allure. Odor is the most primal way of stirring our sexuality, and we are already equipped with the ultimate aphrodisiacs—pheromones, the hormones that humans and most animals secrete in their sweat. Women are particularly sensitive to the sexual lure of androsterone, a pheromone found in the skin and hair of a lucky 10 percent of all men. Many women are also lured by another male pheromone, exaltolide, the source of the musky scent in some perfumes. The female equivalent, "copulins," is a pheromone found in vaginal fluids.

The essential ingredients of today's perfumes are still often related to the sexual function of animals or plants. For example, musk is secreted by the male deer to use as a sex lure. We extract this animal perfume from the appropriate gland in the deer to use in our own perfumes. Even our floral perfumes are related to sexual play. The oil glands of flowers are used to attract insects, thereby promoting the flower's own fertilization.

### *Eastern Use of Scent*

In tantric and Taoist lovemaking, pure essential oil essences are always used, never synthesized scents. Synthesized scents either isolate the elements scientists consider to be most active, excluding other important elements of the flower, or they are simply chemical replications loaded with potentially allergenic substances.

It takes a tremendous quantity of the flower to distill even a tiny amount of a true essential oil, but the benefits in terms of purity and potency make the process more than worthwhile.

The chief reason for using scent in tantra and Taoist lovemaking is to stimulate the root, or first chakra—the energy center located at the base, or sacrum, of the spine—that is considered to be the seat of sexual desire and response. This does not mean, however, that you apply the oil only to the base of the spine. Behind the ears, the inner thighs, breasts, and underarms are also choice spots.

Among the pure oils commonly used by tantric practitioners are musk (greatly diluted as it is very powerful), jasmine oil, patchouli, sandalwood, saffron, vanilla, ylang-ylang, and spikenard. But you can use any essential oil that appeals to you.

### *Finding Your Personal Scent*

A key to using scent to enhance your sex life is to find your own personal scent. Many people are experimenting with aromatherapy—the use of powerful pure essential oils to alter mood, attract the opposite sex, and even heal ailments. Some of these natural extracts from plants and flowers contain chemicals that actually trigger the brain to respond sexually, because the body's smell center is in the limbic system of the brain, the part that also controls emotional and sexual responses. This is why researchers have found that certain scents will set off reactions in the brain areas governing sexuality.

You may find that a single pure scent is perfect for you. Or you can blend several pure essential oils together to create your signature scent.

Pure essential oils are readily available at natural body-care store chains and through countless companies that sell them by mail order. You can experiment by visiting shops that sell pure essential oils—check to make sure their oils are pure—and playing with combinations right on the premises. Or you can purchase samplers by mail order and mix the oils at home.

### *Aphrodisiac Massage*

A light massage combined with the appropriate essential oil or combination of oils is called an aromatherapy massage, and it can be deliciously stimulating to your libido. It is also a great way to begin a sexual encounter. As you receive the massage, inhale deeply to take in the benefits of the oil's aroma.

If you are stressed and frazzled by the pressures of daily life, calming essential oils, such as rose, jasmine, chamomile, neroli, sandalwood, and vetiver will help ease the stress and bring about a calmer state of mind that is more conducive to lovemaking.

On the other hand, if you are fatigued and too tired for sex, try an aphrodisiac massage that uses stimulating oils like peppermint, nutmeg, or tea tree.

Use these oils with discretion. Most cosmetic and beauty products containing essential oils have low enough percentages to be considered safe. The pure essential oils that are readily available through catalogs or at any health food store must be combined with a pure, cold-pressed vegetable oil—such as sesame or sunflower—as a carrier, using no more than twenty drops of pure essential oil per pint of carrier oil. If you bathe in essential oils, use no more than eight to ten drops of oil per tubful of water.

## Aphrodisiac Foods

### *Phosphorous Foods*

Phosphorus-rich foods have been regarded as aphrodisiacs for centuries, because of this mineral's stimulating properties to the sex glands and its strengthening action on the sex organs. Bird's Nest Soup, a staple of Chinese love cuisine, is made from the nest of sea swallows, which contains high amounts of phosphorus. In fact, the whole of Chinese cuisine is designed to enhance sexual desire and performance.

Another love food, truffles, owes its reputation to high levels of phosphorus. This mineral is also present in large quantities in oysters, clams, and east Indian curries, chutneys, and hot sauces—all of which are dubbed aphrodisiacs because their hot spices also mildly irritate the sex organs—just enough to be sexually stimulating.

Eggs and fish are reputed to be sexual restoratives because they contain high quantities of phosophorus. The lecithin in raw egg yolks contains phospholipid, a form of phosphorus that supports hormone gland secretion, tones sex glands, and strengthens nerves. Since male ejaculate is high in lecithin, if phosphorus levels drop, virility sinks too.

Your body needs substantial amounts of phosphorus, and it must work in a specific ratio with calcium. (See chapter 1 for the specific recommended ratio of calcium-magnesium-phosphorus.)

Among the foods that are good nutritional sources of phosphorus, and therefore can be considered aphrodisiacs, are wheat bran, pumpkin seeds, squash seeds, sunflower seeds, sesame seeds, brazil nuts, almonds, walnuts, cashews, peanuts, pinto beans, rye, millet, dulse, kelp, chicken, crab, beef, lamb, lentils, mushrooms, garlic, sweet corn, raisins, yogurt, and brussels sprouts.

### *Celery*

Taken as a food or in herbal form, celery contains the female-luring male hormone androsterone, which, after it is eaten, is then released in sweat. Androsterone also elicits the response of testosterone, which increases libido. Celery is also considered an aphrodisiac because of its high mineral contents, especially naturally occurring sodium.

You can take one celery capsule a day. If you eat the raw stalk, make sure it's not affected by pink rot (you will notice pink and brown spots on the stalks). That means it has a high content of psoralens, which cause sensitivity to the sun's rays.

### *Avena Sativa* (Green Oats)

Oats increase orgasm frequency, boost sex drive, and enhance performance by liberating those all-important sex hormones. You can eat cooked oats (do not use oatmeal in its processed or flake form) or take a pill form of a sex drive–stimulating folk remedy called avena sativa, which is made from green oats.

Excitiva is a popular tablet from Switzerland made from green oats and is recommended by natural health-care providers to enhance male potency and increase female libido.

*DOSE:* One tablet after each meal.

*SAFETY ISSUES:* None

## HERBAL "APHRODISIACS"

Most reputed aphrodisiacs are herbs. They may not be miracle quick fixes for serious problems with your hydraulics, but they will definitely perk up libidos, enhance your ability to perform, and increase sexual satisfaction overall. All of these herbs should be taken prior to having sex.

### *Yohimbe*

This West African tree bark has been proven in early studies to increase sexual desire in women and improve erections in men. In Africa, yohimbe has been smoked, eaten, and sniffed for centuries for its aphrodisiac properties. Here in the West, it has been embraced in recent years by those seeking more frequent, longer-lasting lovemaking. In fact, yohimbe's recent popularity has come about mainly because of the loss of libido experienced by many people who take antidepressant drugs (aka selective serotonin re-uptake inhibitors, or SSRIs). Yohimbe is employed by doctors and sex therapists as a treatment for impotence, especially to counter those libido-squashing effects caused by SSRIs. Medical doctors often prescribe a form of yohimbe (available by prescription only) called yohimbine hydrochloride.

Yohimbe works by dilating the blood vessels, thereby bringing blood closer to the surface of the sex organs. It also increases the excitability of the lower spinal cord, from which branch major nerve bundles that lead to the sex organs and glands. In addition, yohimbe also owes its aphrodisiac properties to its ability to work as a testosterone precursor, thereby increasing levels of the hormone that produces sexual desire. It also lowers blood pressure and builds muscle tissue.

The fluid extract is your best bet because it is more standardized for active properties than capsules and is also the strongest natural form of yohimbe.

---

If you are on SSRI treatment, you might want to try herbal remedies instead (but only under your doctor's guidance!). Damiana is a natural antidepressant as well as a great tonic for the sex organs and glands, and St. John's wort is currently getting wide publicity for its ability to relieve mild cases of depression.

---

*DOSE:* Dose is determined by your body size. If you weigh 150 pounds or less, take no more than five to ten drops in a half glass of water, half an hour to forty-five minutes before you have sex. If you're larger in size, then fifteen to twenty drops, taken a half hour to forty-five minutes before lovemaking, will be enough.

*SAFETY ISSUES:* Yohimbe can increase testosterone in the blood stream, which could predispose some men to prostate cancer and cause some women to grow facial hair. That increase of testosterone blood levels could also cause an increase in blood pressure, disposing some people to hypertension. It also means that those suffering from high blood pressure or heart arrhythmia should not take this root. Some researchers are also looking into the possibility that yohimbe overtaxes the liver and kidneys.

For those who have low blood pressure, using yohimbe as an aphrodisiac can produce the oppposite effect by lowering the blood pressure even further. That means it can cause fatigue, and men can suffer a temporary bout of impotency.

The good news is that a number of recent studies conducted in the United States and Germany found that some of these possible side effects can be countered by taking 1,000 mg of buffered vitamin C in the morning and another 1,000 mg dose in the evening.

Yohimbe should not be taken at the same time as foods or any other substances containing the amino acid tyramine (liver, cheese, red wine, as well as some diet aids and decongestants).

## *Muira Puama* ("Warrior Wood")

This herb from Brazil qualifies as an aphrodisiac because, like yohimbe, it boosts testosterone blood levels, thereby increasing sexual desire and energy levels.

*DOSE:* Muira puama is also best taken in liquid extract form. Follow same instructions as for yohimbe.

*SAFETY ISSUES:* The same warnings given for yohimbe related to high blood pressure and possible masculinization in some women apply to muira puama. Studies have also found that these possible side effects are countered to some extent by taking 1,000 mg of buffered vitamin C twice a day.

### *Kava Kava*

Captain Cook named the plant he encountered in Tahiti "intoxicating pepper," because ancient Tahitians and other South Pacific Islanders used its ground-up roots mixed with either water or coconut water to create a drink that toned the sex organs and glands and stimulated their lovemaking. The drink was also consumed by villagers at their nightly gatherings and at important ceremonies because kava kava is also a powerful herbal relaxant and mood enhancer that gives greater clarity of thought.

The kava kava root's active ingredients are called kavalactones. A recent controlled study in Germany compared a group of patients who took a placebo with those who took 70 mg capsules of kava kava three times a day. All patients tolerated the herb well, with no adverse reactions, and it was found to be effective over both the short and long term.

Kava kava works best as an aphrodisiac if the prospect of sex makes you anxious and hampers your sexual enjoyment. It decreases muscular tension, induces relaxation without a feeling of being drugged, peace and contentment, mild euphoria, sexual receptivity, and increased sociability. It may also increase the size of a woman's clitoris, thus increasing her sexual sensitivity, and has been found to provide temporary relief for menopausal women suffering from anxiety.

When taken in moderate doses, this leaf produces an aphrodisiac effect within half an hour that lasts for a few hours, time enough to squeeze in a steamy lovemaking session.

*DOSE:* To use as a sexual tonic, take one 250 mg capsule after breakfast and one after dinner. If you do not need kava kava as a tonic and just want to use it whenever you have to perform on short notice, take one capsule or ten drops of the fluid extract a half hour before lovemaking. Make sure the brand you choose is standardized to give you a consistent amount of the kavalactones.

*SAFETY ISSUES:* High doses—more than the recommended dose given above—can cause stomach upset or a slight skin rash. This herb has not been studied for years, so at this point it's recommended that you limit use to four months, then take at least one month off. Do not take with more than a small glass of wine or more than six ounces of beer. Do not combine with any sedatives at all.

### *Red Clover*

Red clover blossoms have a mild estrogenic effect that stimulates vaginal lubrication, and recent research suggests that the active ingredient can prevent cancer. Other factors that contribute to red clover's reputation for increasing sexual potency stem from its cleansing and rejuvenating action on all the body's systems.

Though red clover is generally considered a tonic and a cleanser, for use as an aphrodisiac, add two teaspoons of red clover extract to four ounces of red wine. This "love wine" makes a nice compliment to the Eastern Love Ritual.

### *Panax Ginseng*

Its phallic shape is one reason for this root's age-old reknown as an aphrodisiac, but ginseng's reputation is well deserved. Eastern healers have used panax ginseng for over five thousand years to boost energy levels and improve sexual function. Panax ginseng also grows in North America and was used by Native Americans both as a tonic herb and as an aphrodisiac. It acts on the endocrine glands, stimulating the production of testosterone, and, in women, the production of estrogen.

*DOSE:* Choose a brand standardized to contain at least .5 percent ginsenosides. Take one capsule or ten to fifteen drops of the fluid extract in the morning.

### *Deer Horn Extract*

Interestingly, the Deer exercise described in chapter 4 is named after that animal because its horns have been long prized by traditional Asian healers for the concentrated and highly powerful sexual energy the horns are said to store. Extract of deer horn is currently popular among Hollywood folk for its reputed ability to boost well-being, increase mental acuity, harmonize emotions, and enhance the sex drive. Deer horn (or antler) extract (removed painlessly) is a longtime staple in Chinese herbal medicine formulas, probably because its concentrated protein content boosts sexual response.

*DOSE:* Since no studies have been done to determine dose

level or safety, your best bet is to take this substance only at the prescription of a specialist in Chinese herbs.

*SAFETY ISSUES:* Unknown at this time.

### *Aloe Vera*

The aloe vera plant looks like a cactus plant and grows in warm regions. The long leaves of this succulent are filled with a gel that is packed with healthy oils, vitamins, minerals, amino acids, and other sex function–enhancing ingredients. Aloe gel is reputed to be an excellent aphrodisiac for men and somewhat less so for women.

Aloe gel is also an acid remover from the body, which means it acts as a general tonic, supplying the minerals and vitamin C that are so essential to healthy sexual functioning. Men lose a lot of vitamins and minerals when they ejaculate, so aloe vera can help replenish their supply, especially during a period of intense and frequent lovemaking.

*DOSE:* Drink four to six ounces twice a day, mixed with juice or at full-strength.

*SAFETY ISSUES:* If you use the actual leaf, be sure to only use the clear inside gel. Avoid the red-yellowish substance right under the leafy skin. It has powerful laxative properties—not what we're looking for here.

Other herbs and herbal combinations reputed to have aphrodisiac qualities include a tea made by brewing damiana and saw palmetto together. Both are tonic herbs that also increase the sensitivity of the sex organs and protect the urinary and reproductive tracts from irritation. Use one teaspoon of each herb to make one cup of tea. Or you can combine one teaspoon of the extracts with one cup of water. Fenugreek seeds—eaten whole or taken as an extract or tea—support sex organ and gland health and are also said to increase breast size, which some women feel makes them more sexually alluring.

## DANGEROUS APHRODISIACS

The field of aphrodisiacs is wide open for charlatans; this area is a true case of buyer beware. Be wary of any claims made by manufacturers of aphrodisiacs. When it comes to sex-enhancing substances, follow the recommendations made in this book, along with the advice of a qualified expert in natural medicine, because some of these so-called aphrodisiacs can actually be life-threatening.

### *Mandrake Root*

The root of mandrake, a plant in the deadly nightshade family, has a centuries-old reputation as an aphrodisiac. It is also known to be highly dangerous and can cause vomiting, cramps, convulsions, and even death.

Mandrake is unavailable for purchase in any store and even by mail order. If by some wild chance someone offers it to you or you come across a mail-order advertisement, do not—under any circumstances—take it.

### *Spanish Fly*

This powder, prepared from a cantharis beetle, can cause the same potentially lethal symptoms as mandrake root. It is also largely unavailable. One product on the market called Spanish Fly Formula contains no powdered cantharis beetle, but uses cayenne powder, which irritates sensitive mucosa, thereby creating a sensation that is supposed to be sexually exciting.

### *L-dopa*

There have been no studies of L-dopa on women. The drug, which is popular with "smart drug" advocates, is prescribed for Parkinson's disease because it stimulates production of the neurotransmitter dopamine, which plays an essential role in sex drive.

Nonetheless, no studies have been conducted on the efficacy and safety of using L-dopa to enhance sexual response. It is not recommended that you self-administer this prescription drug, which, in any case, cannot be obtained legally for purposes other than treatment of Parkinson's disease.

### *Deprenyl*

This is another so-called "smart drug" that cannot be legally prescribed except for treatment of Parkinson's disease. Deprenyl also increases levels of dopamine, thereby increasing libido and sexual stimulation.

Again, do not use deprenyl as an aphrodisiac, as no studies regarding the safe use of deprenyl for increasing libido have been conducted.

### *Gamma Hyoxybutyrate* (GHB)

This controversial drug is touted highly by its proponents as an aphrodisiac for men and women. It supposedly gives men longer-lasting, harder erections and delays ejaculation and makes the vagina more sensitive, giving women more powerful orgasms and freeing them from inhibitions.

While this may sound good, the drug—initially popular for reducing fat and building muscle—is dangerous, and it doesn't take much to cause severe poisoning. Users are advised never to take GHB with alcohol, tranquilizers, or allergy and sleep medications.

There is so much research that needs to be done before GHB is approved—if ever—that it's safest to stay away from it altogether. In any case, it's difficult to find. In fact, since several headline-making deaths from GHB several years ago, this drug has disappeared from store shelves and can only be purchased in Europe.

### *Viagra*

Viagra is a new drug designed to improve male potency that has become very popular recently, although it is not being touted as an aphrodisiac, but as an adjunct to sex stimulation. Its manufacturers claim that if Viagra is taken one hour before sexual activity, it will restore potency in most men.

Viagra works by inhibiting an enzyme that breaks down a body chemical that causes blood vessel constriction. The result is increased circulation that enables the penis to engorge with blood and become erect. Viagra also prolongs the period of erection. Its manufacturers claim an excellent safety profile and that it was successful on seven out of ten impotent men in their clinical trials.

Although no studies have been done as yet on women, they have begun taking the drug in order to increase blood flow to their sex organs, which potentially increases their sensitivity. Some women who do not even suffer any sexual dysfunction are trying the drug out of curiosity, despite doctors' warnings that no one knows what the long-term effects might be for women.

Viagra's *known* possible side effects are numerous, including headaches, stomachaches, blurred vision, and inability to correctly perceive certain colors. It also cannot be taken by diabetics, those with severe prostate problems, or those who are taking certain cardiac medications, in particular nitroglycerin preparations. Unfortunately, these three groups—diabetics, men with prostate problems, and men with cardiovascular ailments—constitute the overwhelming majority of those who suffer from chronic impotency.

That factor, plus the drug's possible side effects, suggests that the wisest course in treating impotence is still to try all reasonable—and health-supporting—natural solutions first.

Unfortunately, many doctors who prescribe drugs like Viagra or HRT in order to enhance the libidos of their patients are unaware of the many natural options that also enhance overall health and carry less risk of dangerous side effects.

In any case, your safest choice when it comes to aphrodisiacs—and virtually everything else regarding your health and sexuality—is first to explore the options Mother Nature has to offer.

# 11

# NATURAL TREATMENTS FOR COMMON SEXUAL PROBLEMS

As you now know, good physical and mental health are a prerequisite for good sex. The reverse is equally true: We need to make love, not just for our physical well-being but to ensure and protect our emotional and mental health.

Each of us is a unique, interconnected entity made of body, mind, emotion, and spirit. This means that even if a sexual problem originates in an emotional, mental, or spiritual conflict, it can be effectively treated through either the physical body or the mind.

How you use the gift of sex is crucial to your overall well-being. If you suppress your sexuality or are often frustrated with regard to sex, your entire life is affected, and your sense of belonging—to yourself and to the human community at large—suffers. If you don't get help with your sexual problem, it can become chronic and cast a shadow over every other aspect of your experience.

Sexual problems are often self-created. Poor diet, lack of exercise, and chronic stress can lead to disease and dysfunction and set you up for such common sexual problems as impotence, premature ejaculation, inability to orgasm, lack of libido, sexual boredom, and painful intercourse. But these sex-related problems can also be caused by emotional and mental conflict.

## The Most Common Blocks to Sexual Pleasure

The most common blocks to your sexual pleasure are those created by that most powerful of sex organs—your brain. Misbeliefs about sexuality can jam the sexual messages that normally course freely between your brain and groin. As you learned in chapter 7, in order to resolve sexual problems caused by this mental static, you must first discover, then correct your mistaken belief systems and fears. Two of the common sex-related problems that invariably originate in the mind are concerns over penis (and vagina) size and body image.

In addition, we in the West are particularly prone to a relentless performance pressure. The anxiety created by this goal-oriented approach to sex underlies many sexual problems and dysfunctions. When worrying reaches obsessive levels, you lose your ability to let go and immerse yourself completely in the lovemaking experience. You are no longer an involved participant; you become a distanced observer and self critic. This phenomenon becomes self-perpetuating, with your anxiety building and removing you further and further from sexual pleasure, as each "failed" event fuels your concerns.

Nothing dampens sexual desire more than this extreme self-consciousness. In order to surrender to the bliss of sex, you need to be relaxed and comfortable.

Physical weakness and deficiencies can be an equally destructive factor in your sex life. If you want to keep your libido high and enjoy sex, you need to maintain good nutrition, get the right type of exercise, and allow yourself enough rest. You may also need to take supplements and herbs to maintain sexual strength and vigor, especially if you are over thirty and your supply of essential hormones, proteins, antioxidants, and other substances has begun to dwindle. After age thirty is also a great time to begin exploring traditional Eastern solutions to sexual strengthening and healing: acupuncture, acupressure, yoga, and Taoist exercises. These are powerfully effective strategies for both preventing and curing sexual problems.

## OVERCOMING SEXUAL PROBLEMS

The first step in dealing with any sexual problem is to rule out any possible physical disease or dysfunction that requires the attention of a doctor. See a doctor for a thorough checkup to eliminate disease factors. Cardiovascular disease, high or low blood pressure, Lyme disease, hormonal imbalances, diabetes, prostatitis, chronic viral, parasitical, or bacterial infections, and other maladies can rob you of the vitality you need for sexual activity. Low libido, for example, can be a side effect of prescription antidepressants or the result of consuming too much alcohol, tobacco, or recreational drugs.

If you have ruled out the above, the next step should be to look to your health lifestyle: your diet, exercise habits, and how much stress you have to deal with.

### *Diet*

Is your diet high in fast foods, processed foods, sugar, "bad" fats, and simple starches? Are you eating foods that support and nourish sexual function? These include eating more high-fiber foods, such as fruits, vegetables, and grains. Also, cutting down on alcohol, especially beer, keeps your sex glands healthy.

*GRAINS:* Daily servings of whole grains that are free of pesticides supply sex organ and gland-boosting vitamin E and the trace minerals that are essential to optimum sexual function.

*FRUITS AND YELLOW AND GREEN VEGETABLES:* Daily servings give you many of the minerals and vitamins—especially vitamins A and C—you need to promote sexual health.

*FATTY FISH SUCH AS SALMON AND TUNA:* Servings of fatty fish at least four times a week provide enough oils for your body to convert into essential fatty acids, the raw material for sex hormones. These fish are also low in harmful cholesterol.

*FENUGREEK, PUMPKIN, SESAME, AND SUNFLOWER SEEDS:* Regular servings, several times a week as a snack or sprinkled on foods, boost hormone levels and energize and tone the sex organs and glands of both genders.

*SOY PRODUCTS:* Servings at least four times a week for women over forty, who need more estrogen because their body's production of the hormone is dwindling, and women who suffer from PMS, which is often caused by their body producing overly high levels of estrogen. Soy contains safe plant forms of estrogen, which bind to estrogen receptor sites, thereby signaling to the body to lower its production of more harmful forms of the hormone. A diet rich in soy products increases sexual vitality and desire, decreases incidence of PMS, and even lowers the risk of breast cancer, particularly in postmenopausal women who would otherwise take hormone replacement therapy or higher doses of HRT.

*CALCIUM FOODS OR CALCIUM-MAGNESIUM SUPPLEMENTS:* Women over forty need to consume three daily servings of calcium-rich foods or take calcium-magnesium supplements that add up to 1,000 mg of calcium (and half as much magnesium), the minimum recommended dose to prevent osteoporosis. Even if you're in your twenties—a long way off from menopause—it's never too early to stock up on calcium.

*AVOID HYDROGENATED VEGETABLE OILS:* Margarine and fried foods and other hydrogenated vegetable oils interfere with prostaglandin metabolism and can contribute to prostatitis, not to mention cardiovascular disease. The total amount of fat in your diet should amount to no more than 30 percent of your daily caloric intake, and that fat should be unsaturated.

### *Exercise*

Do you exercise at least three times a week? Or do you exercise too often and obsessively, leaving your energy reserves too depleted for sexual activity? As you learned in chapter 4, experts in yoga and Taoist exercises observe that despite America's exercise craze, few Western exercises are designed to increase overall energy or to strengthen and tone the pelvic muscles, as well as improve their flexibility. What also makes these Eastern exercises such wonderful sexual restoratives is that they focus on increasing the energy and function of the sex organs and glands. Without regular practice of these exercises, traditional Asian healers believe that over time and continuous orgasmic discharge, the sex organs and glands lose life-force energy and muscle tone. The sexual region becomes "cold," that is, unfeeling and numb, and sexual desire vanishes. Not only does the sex life suffer; the person grows old and weak before his or her time.

### *Lifestyle*

Do you get enough rest? Are you plagued with worries and stress? If so, practice the relaxation and visualization exercises in chapter 5.

Now, let's examine the most common sexual problems one at a time and explore the natural treatments that help you to resolve them.

## Lagging Libido

Lack of sexual desire and bedroom boredom are the number one sexual complaints today, and the number of people who suffer from these pervasive sexual problems seems to be climbing daily. As is the case with almost any sexual problem, lack of desire can be a symptom of either physical disease or dysfunction or mental or emotional conflict.

Once disease is ruled out, look to chronic fatigue caused by poor nutrition. You need energy for good sex, and if your diet is barely nutritious enough to get you through your day, nighttime lovemaking inevitably suffers.

Consult chapter 1 to check if you are eating the right foods. "Empty," overly processed foods saturated in pesticides and other chemicals and full of sugar and simple starch rob you of the crucial nutrients you need for a healthy sex life.

Make an herbal tonic part of your daily routine. (See chapter 2 for recipes and suggestions.)

Take a daily multivitamin-mineral, plus supplements of the essential chemicals you need if you're over thirty (see chapter 3). You may want to see your doctor to check your blood levels of essential vitamins and minerals. Sometimes all it takes is a month or so of the right diet, plus key supplements, to restore your energy and wake up your libido.

If this bout of sexual sluggishness is temporary, try taking any of the aphrodisiacs described in chapter 10 half an hour to an hour before you have sex. If your problem is ongoing, start a regular daily regime of either a single herb or a compound herbal remedy that will tone and stimulate your sex glands and organs over a longer term (see chapter 2).

Acupuncture and acupressure can help to increase the strength and function of the sex organs and glands in order to revive your sexual interest and libido. See chapter 4 for acupressure points you can stimulate yourself to strengthen your sexual function.

Lack of exercise can lead to chronic fatigue and disinterest in sex. Exercise at least three times a week to maintain high energy levels. You should also make Eastern practices, such as yoga and Taoist exercises, part of your regular routine. Two basic Taoist exercises, the Deer and the Kidney Stimulator, are among the most effective remedies for lack of libido, as well as for treating inability to orgasm, impotence, and premature ejaculation. (See chapter 4 for complete instructions on how to do these and other Taoist exercises.)

### *Psychological Causes*

If your health and energy levels are fine, but you'd rather read a book or watch your favorite TV program than make love with your partner, you've got a case of sexual burnout. Even mild depression can cool you down, as can job stress. Or you may have simply slipped into a lovemaking rut. It's natural for passion between longtime couples to cool from time to time. But if sex has become so routine and predictable that you could phone it in, you need to inject the elements of surprise, intrigue, and fun into your lovemaking. Here are some suggestions:

- Changing the time you usually get together can create a note of variety and newness. For instance, most sex acts occur at home in bed between six p.m. and midnight. Including unexpected lunchtime or any other unusually timed sex adds the fun and excitement of spontaneity.
- Work with your body clock. Track the highs and lows of your overall energy and libido. Put lovemaking at the top of your agenda when you and your partner feel sexiest.
- Use your erotic mind power. Don't allow yourself to feel guilty about your fantasies. If you think he or she would be receptive, share your scenarios. Watch erotic films, read erotic novels, and take note of sexy people around you. Consult chapters 7 and 9 for fantasies, games, and other creative ways to spice up your love life.

• Create new lovemaking rituals. One couple has a fun Sunday morning custom that gives them an invigorating workout at the same time. They put some hot dance music on the stereo, dance nude around the living room with abandon, then make their way into the bedroom, where they collapse on the bed and make passionate, sweaty love.

• Make a list of what turns you on and give it to your partner.

• Surprise your partner. Give him or her an unexpected gift. Dress up at home (or wear something provocative). Make the unexpected romantic gesture—flowers, a love note packed in his or her lunch bag or in the sock drawer. You can create romantic rituals for the two of you.

• Be affectionate, physically and verbally. This helps protect and maintain your passion and intimacy.

• Inject some fun and silliness into your lovemaking. Engage your partner in a tickle fest; a game of hide and seek around the house or the neighborhood! Play tag, chasing each other down the street. Feed each other dessert. Remember to bring that playful approach into the bedroom.

• Eliminate sexual goals. Every sexual encounter doesn't have to last for a certain length of time or always conclude with an orgasm. Simply share the pleasures of being together.

• Be willing to experiment. Try new positions and techniques you may have read about here or in another book, or even seen in an erotic movie. Try making love half-dressed instead of nude. Commit to a new way of making love for a week or so.

Teach each other new sexual techniques and be open about what feels good and what doesn't.

• Don't just undress separately and put your clothes away. Either tear them off each other, or strip each other slowly in the midst of kissing and caressing. Dance nude for each other by candlelight. Do a slow striptease for your partner to sexy music.

• Turn off the TV before you make love. Institute a "no TV" rule for a week and find other, more interesting ways to spend your evenings together.

• File those flannel pajamas in the trash can and don't wear heavy, unattractive creams to bed. Make yourself feel and look desirable.

• Make some noise. Cast aside your self-consciousness and express yourself vocally. Moans, groans, sighs, and loud panting let your partner know that you appreciate what he or she is doing. Talk dirty, unless your partner finds that a turn-off or a distraction.

• Make eye contact. The look in your eyes can be more expressive than any words.

• Blindfold your partner and make love to him or her. Take turns or make love while both of you are blindfolded.

• Give your partner a pedicure.

• Write your partner an erotic poem.

• Write each other sexy letters. Be graphic.

• Have wild phone sex during office hours.

• Make love in the backseat of a car, in the office after hours, or at some other location that adds a thrilling element of risk.

• Have a makeover. Yes, your lover is supposed to love you for the inner you, but if you look and feel out of shape, your sex life will naturally be affected.

• Exercise regularly. (See chapters 4 and 5 for descriptions of specific exercises.) Try working out together. You'll feel much more energetic and sexier if you're in good physical condition.

• Get out of your rut. Are you in your own personal rut as an individual? That will adversely affect your life together as a couple. Try new interests, skills, and hobbies, and you will be able to bring something different, interesting, and new to your relationship.

• Make changes in your life together. Try new restaurants, visit new places, take walks or bike rides. Take turns serving breakfast in bed on weekends.

• Enjoy a sex getaway. Take a weekend trip to somewhere new and private. Make it an opportunity to play some of the games suggested here and in chapters 8 and 9.

• Give each other new pet names and keep them absolutely private—your sweet little secret as a couple. And don't forget to name each other's sex organs.

• Don't bring anger into the bedroom. If you can't let go of resentment for some injury your partner committed against you in the past or a continuing pattern of negative behavior toward you, don't think that anger won't contaminate your sex life together. It is stored in your body and will turn your bed into a battleground. The solution is not sex, but to express your feelings as calmly and rationally as possible, and owning them as yours. Try to share your feelings and concerns, then work on solutions. If this seems impossible, consider relationship counseling or bailing out of the relationship altogether.

## Too Busy for Sex

This is another common complaint, especially among the many modern career men and women who live under constant pressure and stress. The "too busy for sex" syndrome is often tied to chronic fatigue and low libido.

Children, lack of time, work stresses, money problems, tension piling up from all of life's minor and major irritations, are only some of the obstacles that can come between you and your partner and your sex life together. No one who has experienced juggling the demands of career and family would say that finding time for great sex is easy. It isn't.

All of the solutions given above can motivate couples to find more time for sex. The following additional suggestions will help you to rearrange your schedule so that you squeeze in lovemaking time:

- Give yourself permission to be more self-indulgent. No matter how long your list of daily duties, take time for a long walk, a stolen afternoon at the movies, a leisurely, relaxing bath. Once you allow yourself these humble pleasures, you'll be more likely to regularly schedule in the more exotic pleasures of sex.
- Schedule your lovemaking sessions. While you may prefer lovemaking to be spontaneous, in this context it requires that you set aside a certain amount of free time. You simply have to put sex at the top of your priority list and then deliberately create the mood, instead of waiting for the mood to strike.
- Make a regular weekly date with your partner, not necessarily to make love but just to share time together: a cozy dinner for two, an evening in front of the fireplace, a long walk in the woods.

• Take turns giving each other a massage with scented oil or lotion. You can make massage part of your once-a-week date.

• Don't spend every night in front of the TV set or in front of the computer screen. Play a board game together, read, listen to favorite music, even dance together.

• If you don't usually go to bed at the same time, make sure you do go to bed together at least a few nights a week.

• Try to reserve arguments and/or discussions over issues for the daytime. Don't try to make love when one or both of you is still fuming.

• Create rituals to mark the division between your daytime work life and your evening and night life together. It could be ten minutes of Eastern breathing exercises, a relaxation exercise, a visualization, yoga practice, a long bath, a walk, or simply taking a few moments to consciously replace your negative thoughts about work issues with positive thoughts about how you and your partner will share your time together. Try to keep take-home work to a minimum.

• Set your alarm clock for dawn love, which, according to most body clocks, is an ideal time, since testosterone levels are at their peak. Then, drift off to sleep for an hour or so before you start your day.

• Remind yourself that when it comes to lovemaking, it's quality, not quantity, that really counts.

• Take yourself out of your everyday routine with role playing, games, and fantasies. See chapter 9 for inspiration.

• Make sure your children know that your bedroom is your inner sanctum. When the door is closed, they do not enter.

• If life's pressures block your sexual pleasure whenever you do find time to make love, try to become more aware of the stream of worries, fears, and resentments related to work and other responsibilities that runs like a tape loop in your brain. Every time you become conscious of these thoughts in the midst of making love, cancel them out or delete them, as if you were pressing a button on a computer, and turn your attention to the pleasurable sensations of your body's responses. It may be that you need to share your tensions and concerns with your partner before you actually engage in sex.

# Inability to Orgasm

Most studies find that about 10 to 15 percent of American women never experience orgasm, either through lovemaking or masturbation. And of those women who do orgasm—either through penile-vaginal intercourse or through oral or manual clitoral stimulation—the vast majority experience orgasm only sometimes.

When men have chronic difficulty in reaching orgasm, it is called delayed or retarded ejaculation or male orgasmic disorder.

Again, visit your doctor to rule out the possibility of disease. If that is not the case, look to the following possible factors:

***Physical Causes***

• Certain medications, such as antidepressant drugs, lower libido and can cause inability to orgasm. Try switching to the herb St. John's wort, which has been proven effective in mild cases of depression. Damiana also relieves mild depression and stimulates sexual desire at the same time.

If you do need to take an antidepressant drug, try one of the newer drugs, such as Wellbutrin, or take the herb yohimbe to counter the negative effects on your libido and your ability to orgasm.

• You may not be able to orgasm if you're especially fatigued, stressed-out, overindulge with alcohol, or are a recreational drug user. Obviously, if this is your problem, you need to stop drinking and/or taking drugs. Getting sufficient rest is also a must. If stress is your problem, see the guidelines in chapter 5 for tips on how to relax and reprogram your belief systems so that they are more conducive to sexual enjoyment. If you are temporarily ill, postpone sex until you have recovered.

• If your diet is poor, your body lacks the nutrients it needs to build and release a powerful sexual charge. See chapters 1, 2, and 3 for suggestions on foods, herbs, and supplements that supply the nutrients you need for profoundly orgasmic sex.

• If you do not exercise, you will grow out of touch with your body's sensations. Your body also becomes weaker and more rigid, losing the flexibility, sensitivity, and tone it needs to produce a good orgasm. Yoga and Taoist exercises give you strength and flexibility, and, unlike most Western exercises, they increase, rather than deplete, your energy. See chapter 4 for suggestions on specific exercises to enhance the sexual experience and help you to experience orgasm.

- Inability to orgasm can be caused by shallow breathing that prevents you from getting in touch fully with your sexual sensations. Muscular "armor," chronic muscular tensions, can make your torso rigid and depress breathing. This condition also prevents you from naturally executing the fluid hip movements of sexual intercourse that build arousal—literally "pumping" up sexual energy—and lead inevitably to a full body orgasm. See chapters 4 and 5 for Eastern breathing exercises and bioenergetic exercises that deepen breathing and soften muscular armor.
- Inability to orgasm can be due to a lack of or insufficient foreplay, the sexual activity that takes place prior to intercourse.

Try not to think of foreplay as a chore, something that must be done to pave the way for intercourse, the main event. Foreplay is an essential aspect of the entire love experience, a time to be savored as you stoke each other's fires and bring each other to intense arousal. As you have already learned, Eastern lovemaking techniques focus not on having an orgasm but on drawing out the entire experience so that you are continually building up your excitement, taking it down a notch, then building it up again. This type of lovemaking is much more likely to lead to orgasm. And when you finally do let go to your orgasm, it's far more intense, longer-lasting, and satisfying.

Some men mistakenly believe that their penis should be enough to satisfy their lover. If your partner feels this way, talk the matter over and ask if there's any way he can give you what you need without making him feel inadequate. He may not realize that many women are often slower to become aroused than men. Be sure to praise something about his lovemaking that does please you, at the same time making it clear that sex has to be mutually satisfying.

Try the following tips for heating up foreplay:

### Enjoy an Eastern Love Ritual

See chapter 8 for complete instructions. Or you can extract some of the ritual's elements: Set the scene for romance. Dim the lights or turn them off altogether and light scented candles, arrange fresh flowers, and give your lover a single rose bud. Play sexually inspiring music.

### Use Your Mind Power

Any of the visualizations in chapter 5 will help, or create a scenario to suit you. Start thinking about what you're going to do at night during the day, so that by the time you finally get to bed, you are primed and ready. You can share your fantasy or visualization with your lover or send him/her an erotic note or poem that lays it out in exciting and graphic detail.

### Widen Your Sexual Playing Field

Devote your care to his or her other erotic zones. And take your time. Enjoy long, lingering kisses and slow, soft caresses. Start at your lover's toes, and kiss, lick, and suck all the way up his or her body.

### Give Each Other Oral Sex

This will raise both your temperatures. Faith, who had been a virgin until she met Bob, found that whenever he gave her oral sex, intercourse was much more pleasurable and she was able to have an orgasm. If they skipped oral sex, intercourse was not nearly as exciting.

### Experiment with Different Types of Touch

Use your fingertips to graze your partner's pubic hair and skin as lightly as possible. If you have long hair, sweep it up and down and across your lover's body. Or use a feather. Chinese lovers caress each other lightly with the point of a paintbrush.

### EXPERIMENT WITH DIFFERENT RHYTHMS

Arouse your partner, then back off, lightening and slowing your strokes and caresses. Then, speed up and intensify your touch. This plays with the excitement level.

### BE SURE TO PRACTICE THE EASTERN EXERCISES IN CHAPTER 4

They help you increase your sexual energy and give you control over your aroused energy so that you can enjoy a powerful, pleasurable orgasm whenever you want.

### *Psychological Causes*

The inability to orgasm is often psychological—with fear of surrender cited as the most common cause. You could fear either losing control to this intense experience or becoming too attached to your partner.

If surrender is your problem, the only way to deal with this fear is to challenge it. Ask yourself, "What would happen to me if I did let go?" Your answers will reassure you that the most likely outcomes are intensely pleasurable feelings and freedom from your usual inhibitions. If this problem is too severe for you to handle alone or with your partner, seek professional counseling. Bioenergetic therapy is particularly helpful for this problem.

Examine whether or not chronic resentment is stopping you from "letting go" to your partner. You might be having relationship problems, or you could have unresolved issues around the opposite sex or sex in general. This reason is particularly likely to be the culprit if you are able to orgasm through masturbation or oral sex. If so, sharing your feelings with your partner and working together to resolve them should be your first course of action. If that doesn't work, try relationship counseling.

## IMPOTENCE

By middle age, virtually every man will have experienced at least one or two bouts with impotence. Impotency affects about two hundred million men at some point in their lives, but for some it's a chronic problem. Nothing is more devastating to a man than to expect an erection and not be able to "get it up."

Erections begin with the brain responding to sexual stimulation. The brain orders the nerves to send a chemical signal to the blood vessels so they will send blood into the penis, thereby producing an erection. If you are chronically impotent, either the signal is misfiring or the vessels are so blocked that blood can't fill the penile chambers.

In young men, this embarrassing and anxiety-provoking dilemma is usually caused by drinking too much alcohol, extreme fatigue, illness, legal and illegal drugs, stress, and smoking. Correcting those factors usually resolves the problem.

Unfortunately, chronic impotence is almost epidemic in older men today. Experts estimate that 25 percent of men over fifty are impotent, and more and more men in their thirties are experiencing problems with their erections. Yet impotence is not an inevitable accompaniment to the aging process.

Conventional medicine offers a diverse range of interventions for impotency, such as drugs, penile implants, and vacuum pumps—all of which pose a strong risk of side effects. None of these medical interventions address the root causes of the problem. Nor do any of them restore overall mental and physical health and, by extension, sexual function.

## CAUSES

### *Cardiovascular Disease*

One of the primary causes of this particular bedroom disappointment is cardiovascular disease, which is showing up more frequently in younger men because of poor nutrition, lack of exercise, and chronic stress. Eliminate "bad" fats, cut down on dietary fat altogether, and avoid sugars and simple starches. Eat plentiful servings of tomatoes and tomato products, as well as garlic, all of which have been proven in studies to reduce cholesterol and heart disease.

### *Diabetes*

Diabetes impairs the circulation of blood and energy to the extremities, including the penis. The proper diet (no sugars, no simple starches), acupressure and acupuncture, and exercises such as yoga and Taoist exercises, which increase the flow of energy throughout the body, are all very helpful in treating this condition.

### *Prostatitis*

Enlargement and inflammation of the prostate affects half of men over fifty. This condition can be treated more successfully through diet, herbs, and supplements than through prescription drugs.

Eat a healthy diet free of harmful fats, sugars, and simple starches. Make sure to eat zinc-rich foods (see chapter 1 for a list), especially nuts and seeds, because you need more of this essential mineral that ensures healthy testicular function as you grow older.

The herbs pygeum and saw palmetto are particularly effective when working together to reduce prostate swelling and inflammation and restore penile function. Look for supplements that contain both these herbs, plus zinc.

Acupuncture, acupressure, yoga, and Taoist exercises also help tremendously to correct prostatitis and restore function.

### *High Blood Pressure*

Diet is particularly helpful in lowering blood pressure, especially cutting down on salt intake. Yoga, acupuncture, and acupressure, along with the relaxation exercises and visualizations in chapter 5, all help you cope more effectively with stress—a major contributor to hypertension.

### *Prescriptions*

Prescribed medications (especially antidepressants) can restrict blood to the penis. Damiana and St. John's wort are good herbal antidepressants, and yohimbe is frequently prescribed by doctors to counter the libido-lowering effects of antidepressant drugs.

Impotency can also be caused by too much sexual activity or simply having sex during a time when your body lacks sufficient energy. Taoists recommend a period of abstinence for men with impotency problems, until the body is repaired and energy and hormone levels are restored. Unlike Western sex counselors, Taoists advise refraining from any erotic stimulation until there is complete recovery. Avoid ejaculation, eat properly, and practice Taoist strengthening and flexibility exercises. Within the traditional Eastern view, all physical and emotional problems are rooted in energy imbalances, stagnations, and deficiencies. Once proper energy flow is restored, sexual function will naturally recover.

Impotence can be rooted in psychological causes. Even one "failure" can create so much fear of another incidence of impotency that it sets up a self-fulfilling prophecy. Remind yourself that sex is about giving, receiving, and sharing, not your own performance, a stiff penis, or a blockbuster orgasm. If you have a partner, open up and be honest with her. You can reassure your partner that you love to be with her, but that you are having difficulties. Her support can be tremendously reassuring and help you overcome the problem.

## OTHER SOLUTIONS

### *Tonic and Aphrodisiac Herbs*

Try any of the energy and libido-boosting tonic herbs described in chapter 2 and the aphrodisiacs—yohimbe, kava kava, muira puama, panax ginseng, and red clover wine—described in chapter 10.

### *Yoga and Taoist Exercises*

The yoga postures and breathing exercises and Taoist exercises, such as the Deer described in chapter 4, increase and balance energy and strength in the pelvic area and the body and mind overall, thereby restoring penile function. In fact, regular practice of yoga and Taoist sex exercises both prevents and cures impotence.

### *Taoist Hot Bath Technique*

Immerse yourself in a hot bath. Masturbate yourself to erection. When you are fully erect, grab your testicles forcibly, squeeze, and pull them down at least 100 to 200 times. This grabbing and pulling under water increases the pressure and stimulates hormone secretions and sperm production. If you practice this regularly for a period of time, your potency will increase dramatically. Refrain from ejaculation and whatever energy you have lost will be restored.

### *Deer Variation*

This variation of the Deer is prescribed specifically for impotency problems. Sit on the edge of a chair, testicles hanging free. Use the Basic Eastern Breath throughout. Rub the palms together briskly until they are hot. With one hand, cup the scrotum, with the other hand, rub the lower abdomen back and forth for at least 100 to 300 times. As you rub, inhale and contract the anus, perineum, and buttocks. Hold your breath and the contractions as long as you can.

Once you sense a build-up of energy, use your exhalations to visualize moving that energy all the way up the spine to your brain. Then let it flow down the front of the body, healing everything in its path.

### *Taoist Urinating*

To strengthen the kidneys and adrenal glands (which Eastern healers believe control sexual function), stand on your toes whenever you pass urine, making sure the back and waist are straight. Clench the jaw and buttocks and exhale slowly as you try to forcibly discharge the urine. This technique is also a good corrective exercise for premature ejaculation.

### *Kidney Rocking*

Sit on the floor with your legs together, knees bent and hands on knees. Rock backward to a 45 degree angle, then back again to the starting position. Do this movement as many times as you can and repeat the exercise several times a day. This exercise also increases abdominal strength, which Eastern healers view as an indicator of sexual potency.

### *Anal Pump Squeeze*

This prostate stimulator is easy and effective and can be done anytime, anywhere, to build potency, raise energy, and relieve stress and tension. By toning the anal sphincter, you prevent the debilitation that often accompanies aging. A strong, healthy prostate gland and a toned anal sphincter makes for a long, healthy life with plenty of satisfying sex. Make sure to contract your anal muscles tightly.

Inhale through the nose and, as you hold your breath, do Kegel type pumps, making sure you are pulling up the anal muscles. Exhale slowly and relax.

When you've built up a sensation of warm energy, use your mind power to direct that energy up the spine, into the head, and then down the front of the body.

### *Acupuncture and Acupressure*

Acupuncture is as effective in restoring erectile function caused by emotional problems as it is in cases caused by physical problems. A recent study in Turkey found that twenty out of twenty-nine cases of impotency (none of which were due to physical causes) responded successfully to a series of acupuncture treatments. This resounding success makes sense once we understand that acupuncture is based on the theory that disease and symptoms result from blocks in the body's flow of energy. Even if the cause of impotence is psychological, that fear, anxiety, or other stressful emotions weaken and disrupt the energy flow in the heart, spleen, and kidneys—all of which affect energy and blood flow to the penis.

You can also apply acupressure yourself. Use any of the sex organ stimulating points given in chapter 4. And try the following acupressure massage:

### PENILE REFLEXOLOGY MASSAGE

This massage is pleasurable and restores potency. It is also particularly beneficial to overall health, especially the prostate gland.

1. Using the thumb and fingers, begin at the base of the penis and use a circular motion to work your way to the tip and then back to the base.
2. Take hold of the head of the penis with the index and third fingers and use the thumb to make a circular motion as you press gently with the fingers on the head. Do this as many times as you can, making sure you do not ejaculate.

## LOSS OF ERECTION DURING LOVEMAKING

This problem is similar to impotency, since the man is able to get an erection but loses it during the sex act. Virtually all the causes and solutions given above for impotence can be applied to loss of erection during lovemaking.

Again, once you've experienced an erectile failure, you naturally fear that it will happen again. That fear soon transforms into chronic performance anxiety that could actually cause an isolated episode of losing your erection to become a pattern. Each time you lose your erection, the problem snowballs and becomes worse and worse.

Other possible causes include poor nutrition, weakness due to lack of exercise, temporary illness or injury, noise, and any other distractions. If stress, your inner dialogue, or outside elements distract you from sex, focus on your body's sensations or a particularly sexy fantasy.

### OTHER SOLUTIONS

#### *Share Your Feelings*

If you have a partner, share your concerns with her and reassure her that she is as sexually desirable as ever. An understanding partner can provide much helpful support by not becoming insecure about her attractiveness, by showing empathy without acting overly solicitous, and by avoiding in-depth analyses of other problems between you, of the event, or its impact on your relationship. If this is only an occasional problem, she can try oral or manual stimulation to get you erect, but only for a few moments. If she doesn't get quick results, she can switch to showing affection through embraces, kissing, and caressing.

### *Try Relaxation Techniques and Guided Visualizations*

These can be highly effective. Your anxiety about an erection can be reduced by learning how to relax at a given signal and by reprogramming yourself through a positive guided visualization. Try any of the relaxation and visualization techniques described in chapter 5.

### *Focus on the Visuals*

Since men tend to be excited by visual stimulation, make sure the setting is appropriately erotic, ask your partner to wear something particularly provocative, and focus on the sexual excitement that registers on her face.

### *Activate Your Anal/PC Locks*

Practice the Taoist Energy Transformation Exercise. This gives you so much strength and control over your sexuality that you can will an erection with only the power of your mind.

You can activate your locks during sex to keep your erection strong. Or you can ask your partner to stimulate a harder erection by flexing her PC muscles.

Practice delaying orgasm when you masturbate through the Taoist Energy Transformation exercise or by lightening your strokes as your approach orgasm until your excitement level lowers. Then build it up again. Keep doing this to build up your arousal and keep your penis from wilting.

### *Change Your Method of Stimulation While Making Love*

This also enables you to control your arousal level, building it and taking it down a few notches, while still maintaining a strong erection. Change positions and activities, even vary the ways in which you thrust during intercourse. Try the Taoist nine shallow, one deep stroke pattern.

## PREMATURE EJACULATION

Premature ejaculation occurs when a man ejaculates before or soon after penetration (three to five minutes), with minimal stimulation. A common problem among young men, premature ejaculation is rarely due to a physical problem, although "coming too soon" can become a lifelong pattern.

Just like any erectile problem, chronic stress and anxiety can turn performance fears related to premature ejaculation into a self-fulfilling prophecy. On the other hand, some experts believe that men and women have a "preset" orgasmic threshold. That means that some men reach orgasm quickly, as do some women, but in women, this is not considered a problem.

Eastern sex techniques and exercises are almost entirely focused on delaying the male orgasm! Practice the ones described in chapters 4 and 8, and you will gain a degree of control you never believed possible over your erection and orgasm.

## PAIN DURING INTERCOURSE (MEN)

Sometimes the skin on the man's penis feels raw from friction during sexual intercourse. A certain degree of friction is necessary for sex to be pleasurable, but too much can take your penis out of action for a while.

Your first step should be to consult your health-care provider regarding the possibility of infection. Once those factors are eliminated, the possible causes of your discomfort can range from insufficient lubrication to excessive rubbing on certain sensitive spots to allergies (latex rubber is a common culprit) that cause your genital tissue to inflame and become overly sensitive.

Make sure both of you are lubricated prior to intercourse. Keep a tube of a sex lubricant such as Astroglide, K-Y Jelly, or Sylk on hand.

Also, know your own body. If you tend to become sore in a specific place, vary your angles and positions.

Slowing down can help, as can trying something different. The woman can lie still while you take your time, moving as slowly as you can inside her. Concentrate on your breathing, slowly moving all the way in and all the way out. This approach protects your sensitive areas and might even increase the intensity of your orgasm. In any case, it can't hurt to experiment.

## Pain with Intercourse (Women)

Painful intercourse tends to be a bit more complicated in women because this problem can be caused by many possible physical disorders, emotional factors, or a combination of both. In the majority of cases, though, discomfort or pain during intercourse or upon penetration is usually the sign of a physical disorder, even if your doctor is telling you "it's all in your head."

### PHYSICAL CAUSES

The possible physical causes are numerous. They include vaginal infections and STDs, vaginal dryness (which could be caused by antidepressants, allergy medications, birth control pills, or menopause), bladder infections, vaginal cysts, endometriosis, back pain, and allergic reactions to latex rubber (condoms).

If neither lack of lubrication nor medication is to blame, see your gynecologist to rule out such serious physical causes as endometriosis (a fairly common condition in which the uterine lining grows outside the uterus), ovarian cysts, adhesions (an overgrowth of scar tissue following surgery or infection), pelvic inflammatory disease (commonly caused by a microbe, chlamydia), or, more rarely, a tumor. Get a culture to rule out a strep infection of the vagina, which comes from the same bacteria that causes strep throat and can be passed to you by your partner through oral sex. If this is the problem, penicillin will clear it up.

If medication is causing your vagina to become overly dry and making intercourse painful, consider an herbal antidepressant such as St. John's wort or damiana, or continue your medication and take an herbal boost for your libido in order to counteract those effects. See chapters 2 and 10 for descriptions of herbal choices.

If the problem is lack of foreplay, the solution is evident. If it's vaginal dryness, an over-the-counter, water-based lubricant is an effective remedy, especially if low estrogen levels or a hormonal imbalance is causing vaginal tissues to thin and/or dry out.

If you have developed a thinning of the vaginal mucosa from birth control pills, switch to another means of birth control. If you are menopausal or postmenopausal, use a natural hormone cream such as ProGest locally on vaginal tissues, hormone replacement therapy, and/or any of the natural alternative solutions to low hormone levels described in the next chapter.

Avoid hot tubs and strong deodorant soaps. They dry vaginal tissues, which can lead to further irritation and pain during intercourse.

You could also have a low-grade vaginitis, which causes the vagina to feel irritated during intercourse. Vaginitis can be alleviated by salt water baths, in which one half cup of sea salt is mixed into a full bath. Soak for fifteen minutes, occasionally abrading the vagina and filling it with the water.

Check with your health-care provider regarding allergies to barrier birth control devices—especially those made of latex rubber—and to spermicides. This is a far more common cause of pain during sex for women than many people realize, including doctors.

Sometimes the reasons for pain with intercourse can be persistently elusive. Yoga and the Taoist exercises in chapter 4 are amazingly effective in such cases, because they restore general sexual health and strength, thereby relieving a host of nagging, often mysterious problems that can make sex uncomfortable.

## PSYCHOLOGICAL CAUSES

Psychological causes include stress, early physical or psychological abuse, guilt about sex, fear of sex or intimacy, anger, deep unresolved conflict with a partner, and ambivalence about sex or the relationship.

## PREVENTING VAGINAL INFECTIONS

Minimize the risk of vaginal infection caused by bacteria, fungi, and even viruses, by making your vagina an unwelcome hostess to undesirable microorganisms. In the healthy vagina, bacteria called lactobacilli break down glycogen primarily into lactic acid, which keeps the environment stable and healthy. When this process is disturbed, the way is cleared for yeast and bacterial invaders to flourish. Factors that can upset the delicate vaginal ecosystem include:

*Overuse of antibiotics.* Only take them when necessary, for serious infections. Restore a healthy, balanced urogenital ecology by eating a cup of organic yogurt every day.

*Uncontrolled diabetes.* Follow your health-care provider's dietary guidelines. Avoid sugars and simple starches.

*Hormonal changes* caused by pregnancy, use of oral contraceptives, or hormone replacement therapy. Again, a daily cup of organic unflavored yogurt can help restore "good" bacteria. Switch to a different method of birth control, or an herbal remedy and/or supplement regime to increase and harmonize your hormonal secretions.

*Chronic candida overgrowth.* Candida is a form of yeast that can disturb healthy vaginal ecology. This condition is sometimes alleviated by eating five ounces of organic unflavored yogurt. But if the problem is severe, the candida will feed on the yogurt. In such cases, eliminate sugar (including fruits) and simple carbohydrates—candida's favorite nourishment—from your diet and see a specialist in candida to correct your condition.

*Tampons and sanitary napkins* containing deodorants and other chemicals. Avoid scented toilet paper, tampons, and sanitary napkins. Your local health food store sells unbleached toilet paper, tampons, and sanitary napkins. Or you can order these products from a mail-order catalog (see Resource Guide).

*Prolonged retention of a diaphragm or tampon.* Remove as soon as instructions direct.

*Synthetic fabrics and chemicals* in underwear, tight panties, panty hose, and jeans can increase heat and moisture, thereby encouraging the growth of unwelcome microbes. Even cotton pantie liners can be a problem, because manufacturers saturate the material in harsh, deodorizing chemicals out of the belief that women need to mask the natural smell of their bodies. Instead of subjecting yourself to these harmful materials, wear natural, unbleached cotton panties whenever possible. See Resource Guide for mail-order sources. Or wear no panties at all.

*Improper bathroom habits.* Wipe from front to back after using the toilet and wash the anal opening with mild soap and water after bowel movements. Every month or so, take a salt water bath every day for one week. Use one-half cup of sea salt per tubful of water. Soak for fifteen minutes, abrading your vagina with a finger and occasionally "sucking" the water in, then expelling it.

---

The problem can sometimes be resolved with the help of a loving and understanding partner. If it seems too severe to handle alone or with your partner, consider seeking professional psychotherapy, either for you or you and your partner, especially in cases of severe pain, such as when attempts at vaginal penetration cause an involuntary spasm of the vagina or chronic discomfort.

## Negative Body Image

You may not be enjoying the quality sex life you desire because of issues concerning your attractiveness. This problem is especially common among, but certainly not limited to, women.

Whether you're a male or female, if you are overly self-conscious about your body because you have negative beliefs regarding your physical attractiveness, it is virtually impossible to involve yourself fully in lovemaking. You're constantly distracted by worries about how you look to your partner. If you suffer from a particularly severe negative body image, you may even go so far as to avoid sex altogether in order to preclude the possibility of rejection.

Ironically, feeling sexy, as opposed to looking sexy, is what makes you most desirable. Perfect breasts and cellulite-free thighs or rock-hard abs and bulging biceps are not as powerful turn-ons as an open and enthusiastic sexual attitude.

### HOW TO OVERCOME NEGATIVE BODY IMAGE

The first step in overcoming any problem is to acknowledge that you suffer from it. In other words, you must realize that the problem is not those extra twenty pounds, that you can't afford breast or pectoral muscle implants, or that you don't visit the gym often enough to build yourself a perfect body. The problem is your self-rejection.

If you have a partner, discussing it with him or her can be a great relief. And if your partner can reassure you that he or she finds you attractive, this will take you a long way toward overcoming this obstacle.

Also, give yourself the same counsel you would give a friend. Positive, commonsensical self-talk can bring your self-expectations down to earthly reality. Realize that our society has set impossibly high beauty standards. Remember, even supermodels and actresses have to be enhanced through digital photography techniques, and they have an army of beauty experts and cosmetic surgeons at their disposal.

Remind yourself that men in most societies around the world appreciate, even adore, full-figured women. Full thighs, a rounded belly, and a big bottom are the height of sexual femininity for these men, who would turn up their noses at a waif-thin fashion model.

On the other hand, a little self-improvement can't hurt. A certain amount of vanity reflects a healthy pride in one's self. Lose a few extra pounds and tone those flabby areas—not for others, but for you, in order to feel stronger, more energetic, and a little better about how you present yourself to the world.

Dress to flatter yourself in your daily life, and don't forget to wear a tantalizing little something to bed.

You could use the relaxation techniques and guided visualizations in chapter 5 to ease your anxiety and to "reprogram" your attitudes and beliefs about your body and your sexuality. One simple visualization for negative body image involves confronting the problem directly.

### *Mirror Exercise*

Strip naked and stand in front of a full-length mirror. Closely inspect yourself from every angle. Take your time, about fifteen minutes. If any negative judgments come up, say, "Cancel, cancel," as if you were deleting them from a computer's memory, and then let them go. At the same time, stroke and caress your body, noting how smooth your skin is and how nice it feels. Keep doing this exercise daily, until the impulse to criticize your looks begins to fade and you enjoy your self-caresses more.

If you still can't refrain from negative criticisms, try this exercise in the dark, while lying in bed. Just stroke your body, as you note the silkiness of your skin. Tell yourself how lucky anyone would be to lie next to you.

If this sounds ridiculous and makes you laugh, fine. Wouldn't you rather laugh than be mired in misery over your cottage cheese thighs? Do this exercise often enough, and you'll come to see your body in a newer, more positive light.

If your fears stem from early negative conditioning about sex and your physical appearance from family or religious influences, seek out an authority—an older role model or religious leader—who can "give you permission" to enjoy your body and your sexuality. In general, if this issue is too difficult to tackle alone, professional counseling should be your next step.

## Organ Size and Disparate Organ Size

Some people claim that size doesn't count, that good bedroom technique can override any possible deficiency: "It's not the size of the boat," they say. "It's how it rides the waves."

A recent study suggests that hoary adage is not completely accurate. While it's true that the most sensitive part of the vagina is the first third, which makes penis length relatively unimportant, many women report that they crave the sensation of being completely filled by a man. In fact, most women, and a smaller majority of men, state that size does count after all. That is, that larger, thicker penises are preferred by most women. And although the woman's size is less of a concern to men, surveys indicate that men prefer smaller, narrower vaginas.

No matter what the size of their penis, most men fear that other men's penises are larger than theirs. If this is your concern, don't judge by what you see in the locker room. Many penises are small when flaccid, but double or more in size when erect. And the opposite is also true: large penises are often relatively the same size when fully erect. What many men also fail to realize is that most women report that girth is more important to them than length.

However, size is never important enough to drive anyone to extreme and dangerous measures.

Some plastic surgeons augment penises with fat and collagen injections, and it's not unusual for women to request vaginal tucks after childbirth. But these surgical shortcuts—especially those performed on penises—can cause horrific side effects. It's far wiser, safer, and sometimes even more effective to seek out natural treatments instead.

Remember, sexual passion is much more than the movement of body parts. It is the building up and sharing of energy between a man and a woman that creates, increases, and sustains excitement. And we must never forget that all-important factor: the quality of the relationship, the love and trust between partners. As is the case with virtually any sexual problem, a loving and sensitive partner who makes it clear that he or she appreciates your sexuality can accomplish wonders in helping you overcome concerns about size.

Occasionally, though, it does happen that a man and a woman do not have compatibly sized sex organs. To paraphrase the *Kama Sutra,* an elephant should not mate with a flea. Generally speaking, a small vagina will stretch, over time, to accommodate a large penis. And there are several methods a couple can use to compensate for the match between a small penis and large vagina.

- The woman can practice the Kegeling and Taoist exercises in chapter 4 to tone her vaginal muscles and tighten them at will. She can Kegel during intercourse to make the penile-vaginal contact tighter and turn up the friction.
- During penetration, the man can press his pelvis against the orgasmic crescent described in chapter 7 in order to stimulate the entire area. (Remember, most of the clitoral tissue lies below the skin surface.) If he also "winds his waistline"—that is, makes the pelvic bump and grind motions described in chapter 4—the diffuse pressure and stimulation, especially to the inner vaginal labia and the clitoris, will increase.
- Experiment with other coital positions. In a particularly ef-

fective position that compensates for differences in size, the woman lies on her back and brings her knees to her chest. If she is on her hands and knees, she can drop to her elbows. The man enters from behind and then manually stimulates the woman's clitoris at the same time that he's penetrating her. Or the woman can stimulate herself.

If you are still determined to enlarge your penis size, try the following rather esoteric Eastern exercise that claims to yield actual measurable results.

### *Taoist Penis Enlargement**

This thorough penis massage is accompanied by breath control and visualization. It is supposed to add an inch or more to penis length after only a month or so of regular practice.

1. Inhale through the nose and into your throat, then swallow the air, visualizing it as a ball you are pushing down into your abdomen.
2. After the ball has reached your lower abdomen, "push it" into your penis, at the same time that you press three middle fingers against the perineum, the midpoint between the anus and the scrotum.
3. Breathe normally as you continue pressing against the perineum and use your other hand to pull your penis back and forth in a smooth, rhythmical motion. Do this for a few minutes.
4. Now, massage the shaft of your penis with your thumb and forefinger, using small circular motions, until it's erect.
5. Circle the penis at the base with your hand, then slide the hand forward about an inch at a time, helping to retain vital energy in the penis and making sure that energy goes all the way to the tip.
6. Next, pull your penis to the right and rotate it several times clockwise and counterclockwise.
7. Do the same to the left.
8. Lightly tap each thigh with the erect penis several times.

After you finish this exercise, soak your penis in warm water for a minute or so to help it absorb the energy you've generated.

*Adapted from *Taoist Secrets of Love: Cultivating Male Sexual Energy* by Mantak Chia and Michael Winn (see Resource Guide).

# 12

# GREAT SEX AFTER FIFTY: IT'S NOT OVER TILL IT'S OVER!

The major obstacle to good sex for older people is negative attitudes about sex and aging. Sadly, many people in America fear aging because our society equates sexual attractiveness with youth. Our culture is particularly hard on women, but men—for whom gray hair and wrinkles can be a badge of distinction—are also prey to fears that aging automatically means a loss in sexual potency.

Yet sexual passion doesn't have to end. In fact, sex after fifty can be the most satisfying of your life. If you are a healthy man, there's no reason why you can't enjoy an active, satisfying sex life into your sixties, seventies, eighties, and even beyond. Though your response patterns slow down, you can still achieve and maintain erections. They may not be quite as firm as those of your youth, but they will be hard enough to give you and your partner much pleasure. When you were young, you were probably overly preoccupied with "getting" your orgasm. Age blesses you with the rewards of patience and taking your time.

One of nature's few kindnesses to older women is that they tend to be more orgasmic and self-accepting. Another is that as male response slows down, women's speeds up, so you and your partner are more in sync and foreplay lasts longer. Finally, older men tend to soften up, emotionally speaking. In their later years, they often want the warmth and closeness of sex that most women have craved all along.

As always, health and sexuality are closely interrelated.

Physically, you reap in your senior years whatever you've sown in your younger years. If you are a man who did not get regular exercise, ate non-nutritious foods, and overindulged in alcohol and caffeine, you cannot expect to enjoy good health and sexual vigor after fifty. And if you've been a smoker, you may now pay the price. These are the very same factors that can make a woman's menopausal years and beyond a time of suffering, instead of a period of self-acceptance and peace.

Low libido and impotence in men, and vaginal atrophy and osteoporosis in women are not inevitable accompaniments to the aging process. All the guidelines regarding diet, natural supplements and herbs, exercise, and mind power that you've read about in this book are designed to protect your health and ensure lifelong sexual function so that all your years, including your mature ones, are golden.

This chapter takes a closer look at the particular health and sex issues and problems typically encountered by men and women over fifty. It offers specific natural remedies—foods, herbs, supplements, and exercises—for prevention and treatment. If age-related sex problems do crop up during this time of your life, you have all the information you need to make the right choices from the safest, more effective natural options available.

## AGING AND MEN

Many men are typically concerned about sexual potency, and, as they age, their fears usually increase. They want to have the same energy and endurance they had in their teens and twenties. Although sexual function does change in the later decades of life, there is no reason why "senior" sex can't be as satisfying and exciting as "junior" sex. The majority of healthy older men are able to reach orgasm, but if a man goes too long without an erection, he may lose the ability to have one.

Yet we cannot discount the reality that, according to the latest findings, 25 percent of men over fifty are impotent. That figure could get higher, as more and more men in their thirties continue to experience problems with their erections, in part because of poor nutrition, lack of exercise, a polluted environment, and chronic stress. The primary physical causes of impotency in older men are cardiovascular disease and other circulatory problems, enlarged prostate, and diabetes. Yet all of these conditions can be treated through natural means.

## MALE MENOPAUSE, POTENCY, AND PROSTATITIS

Strictly speaking, the term "menopause" does not apply to men, because they do not experience a universal shutting down of the ability to procreate, as do women. However, many older men experience a decline in virility that corresponds to a decline in their production of testosterone and other body chemicals. Some European researchers refer to this as the "viropause." But this phenomenon is more gradual than female menopause; it doesn't necessarily affect the ability to procreate, and it does not happen to all men.

The term "male menopause" has been used more often and increasingly in this country to describe a pattern of behavior that is also sometimes referred to as the "male midlife crisis." This crisis is usually set off when a middle-aged man experiences erectile difficulties and responds by acting out his denial of aging. In the stereotypical situation, he leaves his middle-aged wife for a much younger woman and starts a second family. (Of course, with today's equality between the sexes, that scenario is not limited to men. Sometimes it's the woman who denies her aging and seeks out new, much younger partners.)

This male "crisis" is often traceable to issues of self-esteem. His appearance has changed, and he fears that his physical attractiveness is gone. If he's also encountered a bout or two of impotency, all this can be deadly to his libido. Nor surprisingly, he may even feel inclined to give up sex altogether.

### *How to Deal With Male Menopause*

If you are in a good relationship, talk over your concerns and fears with your partner and avoid projecting the "blame" from yourself and your own issues onto her. That's all too easy to do, and it's the main reason why men take the short-term, "easy" solution of scrapping their mate and seeking out the thrill of a newer partner. (That thrill often proves transient, leaving the man back at square one.)

If you do work on solutions with your partner, your intimacy should increase and your bond together grow stronger.

Accept that all change isn't bad. Older men take more time in bed, a quality many women seek out in a lover. They also have the years of experience and know-how that enables them to better please their partners. Indulge in longer, more sensual foreplay. This is a great time to explore fantasies and new ways of touching each other. Read chapters 6, 7, 8, and 9 for detailed suggestions.

Alcohol, fatty foods, heavily sugared and/or starchy fast foods, too much caffeine, and smoking add considerably to your risk of physical problems and impotency. Chapter 1 gives you all the information you need to follow a sex-healthy diet. Here are some additional nutritional tips that are particularly important for aging men and women.

- Include frequent servings of omega-3 fatty acids, found in tuna and salmon, which support sex gland function and lower LDL cholesterol and triglyceride levels, thereby helping you maintain a healthy heart and good circulation—essentials for a good sex life. Avoid hydrogenated, or "bad," fats.
- Eat plenty of zinc-rich sunflower, pumpkin, and sesame seeds to keep hormone levels high and balanced and to protect your prostate against BPH, or enlarged prostate.
- Eat freely from chapter 1's lists of foods high in vitamins E, A, C, bioflavonoids, and B complex, as well as foods high in phosphorus, calcium, magnesium, iron, and, most important, zinc, to protect prostate function.
- Eat tomato products. The *Journal of the National Cancer Institute* reports that lycopene, which gives tomatoes their red color, reduced the risk of prostate cancer by nearly 45 percent in a group of men who ate at least ten servings a week of tomato-based foods.
- Take herbal tonics. Before you rush to your doctor to get a prescription for testosterone supplements or Viagra, the "miracle" potency drug (that carries with it the possibility of several dangerous side effects), consult chapter 10 for lists of aphrodisiac herbs to take before you have sex. See chapter 2 for tonic herbs that should be part of your everyday diet in order to protect your prostate and ensure your potency.

The following herbs are particularly helpful to male sexual health:

### Burdock Root (Arctium Lappa)

The leaves, seeds, stalks, and roots of the burdock root make a great tonic for adrenal function, which, in turn, keeps the sex organs and glands in both sexes toned and healthy. Burdock root also helps reduce the size of an enlarged prostate gland and relieves urinary dysfunction. Cooked burdock root makes a delicious, energy-boosting addition to the diet. The Japanese and people who follow a macrobiotic diet boil the roots in salted water and eat them with sauce. You can steam or sauté burdock and eat as much as you want. Burdock root can be purchased at some health food stores and Asian groceries.

*DOSE:* Burdock capsules and extracts are widely available in health food stores. The standard dose for the fluid extract is ten to twenty drops in water per day; follow bottle label instructions for capsule doses. You can also drink the tea freely.

*SAFETY ISSUES:* None.

### Gingko Biloba (Gingko Biloba)

Since blocked blood vessels are a common cause of weak erections, particularly in older men, this blood vessel dilator and toner is a promising natural solution for impotency caused by poor circulation.

*DOSE:* Gingko biloba comes as a standardized fluid extract, at 24 percent potency, and in capsule form. Take ten drops after each meal or one 60 mg capsule in the morning and one in the evening.

*SAFETY ISSUES:* If you are allergic to gingko, you could experience a mild skin rash. Other possible side effects, which are harmless, are increased warmth in the extremities, a slight flush on the skin, or a tender headache. These result from increased oxygen and blood circulation.

Do not take gingko biloba if you have been diagnosed with a blood-clotting disorder. Gingko leaf extract is quite safe. However, ingesting or touching the fruit pulp can cause such side effects as vomiting, diarrhea, headaches, and itchy skin irritations.

## Panax Ginseng

Anecdotal evidence suggests that panax ginseng increases testosterone production more effectively than hormone injections. In animal studies, this root has increased testosterone levels while decreasing prostate weight, which suggests it can reverse impotency and reduce swelling of the prostate gland.

Ginseng is best taken in the morning because of its stimulating action. Various roots differ widely in their effectiveness. Generally, the more expensive the root, the more effectively it works with less risk of irritation. Whole, dried, ginseng root is available at Asian herb stores, health food stores, and through mail order. You can either chew the root, drink the tea, take the powder or mix it in your food, take the fluid extract or swallow capsules.

*DOSE:* Select a brand of capsules standardized to give you at least .5 percent of ginsenosides. Take one capsule a day.

*SAFETY ISSUES:* None for men.

## Pygeum (Pygeum africanum)

Fifty percent of men over forty will develop prostatitis. Ten percent of them will go on to develop prostate cancer, and one-quarter of those will die from it.

There is evidence that pygeum is effective at shrinking enlarged prostates by preventing cholesterol from accumulating there, especially in the early stages of prostatitis (BPH). Although saw palmetto performs some of the same healing actions as pygeum in treating BPH, when they are combined and zinc is added, the result is an even more effective remedy to counter prostate problems and maintain a healthy libido.

*DOSE:* The usual dose is 100 to 200 mg a day of the extract, divided into two or three doses. Look for capsules or tinctures that combine pygeum with saw palmetto and zinc.

*SAFETY ISSUES:* None, except for occasional side effects of nausea and gastrointestinal irritation.

**SAW PALMETTO (SERENOA REPENS)**

Saw palmetto is used increasingly today to prevent and treat BPH. Many studies have confirmed that saw palmetto extract shrinks enlarged prostates and relieves the symptoms of BPH more effectively than does Proscar, the standard prescription drug used for this condition. In fact, in one study, saw palmetto proved effective in nearly 90 percent of BPH patients, usually in a period of four to six weeks.

Over twenty double-blind, placebo-controlled studies have demonstrated that the fat-soluble extract of the berries standardized to contain 85 to 95 percent fatty acids and sterols is effective in relieving all of the major symptoms of BPH. Again, saw palmetto is particularly effective when used in conjunction with pygeum and zinc. In recent years, a few companies have come out with tinctures and capsules that contain both herbs as well as zinc.

*DOSE:* One 80 to 200 mg capsule after each meal. Make sure the capsule is standardized to give 85 to 95 percent of fatty acid sterols. You can also take the equivalent amount of a fluid extract. See bottle label for dose. Again, look for a compound preparation that also contains pygeum and zinc.

*SAFETY ISSUES:* None.

## *Other Helpful Herbs*

Men also benefit from damiana, echinacea, Siberian ginseng root, garlic, ginger root, and sarsaparilla.

Fast-acting aphrodisiac herbs that are taken half an hour to forty-five minutes before having sex include yohimbe, kava kava, and muira puama. See chapter 10 for instructions on their use.

Some compound tonics described in chapter 2 are specifically formulated to boost male sexual function. They include the Damiana and Saw Palmetto Aphrodisiac Tea (half a cup three times a day), Pygeum and Saw Palmetto Tea (three to four cups a day), and American Indian Ginseng Combination Tea (one cup three times a day, or as needed).

## *Supplements*

Even if you are eating a perfectly healthy diet, since your supply of certain essential body chemicals lowers with age, make sure that you are meeting your daily vitamin and mineral quotas. If you are not sure, have your vitamin and mineral blood levels evaluated to pinpoint any serious deficiencies, especially of zinc. Supplement whatever is needed, following the guidelines given in chapter 3.

Among the nutrients you should probably supplement are:

### VITAMIN E

Between 800 and 1,000 I.U.s a day helps maintain hormone production and balance.

### ZINC

60 mg a day helps the thymus gland keep on manufacturing hormones called thymosins, which, in turn, stimulate production of neurotransmitters and sex hormones. Zinc not only helps sperm production; it protects the prostate gland from prostatitis and prostate cancer.

Zinc is particularly essential for production of the male hormone testosterone. As we age, our zinc levels decline. If you smoke, drink alcohol and/or coffee, suffer from infections, or take certain medications, you are also losing zinc and are putting yourself at risk for low testosterone levels. This will cause lowered libido, impotency, and overall weak sexual functioning in both sexes. More and more natural health-care providers blame low zinc levels for inflammation and swelling of the prostate gland (prostatitis or BPH), a near-epidemic condition affecting men over forty, and insufficient vaginal lubrication in mature women. Low zinc level is also thought to be the cause of low sperm count and poor development of the penis and testes. While zinc supplements are often prescribed for all those conditions, your best bet is to protect yourself with dietary sources of zinc.

### BORON

6 mg three times a day helps counter the less obvious symptoms of male menopause.

### Calcium

1,000 to 1,500 mg a day along with half that amount of magnesium, taken at bedtime, is essential to maintain bone density and health, even in men. Also take 400 I.U. of vitamin D to promote absorption of osteoporosis-fighting calcium, especially if you don't get daily doses of sunshine (thirty minutes of exposure on face and arms a day year-round in warm climates; from April to October in temperate zones). Do not worry about calcium supplementation leading to stone formation. In fact, there is evidence that people at risk for kidney stones can decrease their risk by eating *more* calcium.

### Gamma-Linolenic Acid (GLA)

The essential fatty acids are key to keeping the sex glands young, protecting their function, and maintaining hormone output. Take one or two tablespoons per day of cold-pressed flaxseed oil either alone or drizzled on your food. Or you can take a supplement containing a mixed EFA complex to get a balance of Omega 3s, 6s, and 9s. Take one capsule in the morning and one in the evening. All brands give you 500 to 1,000 mg per capsule.

### Glutathione

Some experts believe that glutathione levels decline with age and that low levels of this antioxidant also may be associated with heart disease, arthritis, and Type II, or adult-onset, diabetes. Supplement this important antioxidant to ensure your energy stays high and to protect sexual function. Take between 1,000 to 3,000 mg per day in divided doses.

### Melatonin

Melatonin is commonly touted as a powerful antioxidant that helps regulate the body's clock. It was first touted as a miracle sleep aid because it causes sleepiness in response to darkness. More recently, this pineal gland hormone—aka "the mother of all hormones," because it is a precursor to many of the body's hormones—has emerged as an anti-ager, reputed to have powerful antioxidant and sex-enhancing properties. Some experts say that as we age, free radicals destroy melatonin-making cells in the pineal. Studies show that people over sixty-five have only one-fourth the melatonin levels of twenty-five-year-olds, causing declining immune function, sleep disturbances, and possible increased susceptibility to cancer. Melatonin is also thought to bolster immunity against cancer and infectious diseases, increase energy levels, and recharge flagging libidos.

Walter Pierpaoli, Ph.D., of the Biancalana-Masera Foundation for the Aged in Ancona, Italy, transplanted melatonin-making pineal glands from young mice to old and vice versa. The younger animals died prematurely while the older mice lived 33 percent longer.

*DOSE:* The recommended dose for melatonin as a sleep aid, which is available over the counter, is 2 to 3 mg at bedtime.

*SAFETY ISSUES:* Unknown at this time. Do not exceed recommended dose level for sleep.

## Superoxide Dismutates (SOD)

SOD is an antioxidant nutrient that prevents the sexual apparatus from aging prematurely because of the action of free radicals. Free radicals invade cell membranes and cut off their oxygen supply.

Some experts believe that SOD's anti-inflammatory properties stabilize cell membranes, thereby retarding aging and allowing you to enjoy youthful desire and passion longer.

*DOSE:* SOD should be taken with manganese, $B_6$, zinc, and magnesium because they are cofactors for the efficacy of SOD. If you're already taking a multiple mineral, you do not need to supplement the above cofactors individually.

Take one 2,000 unit of SOD in a tablet labeled "enteric-coated" (which means it bypasses your intestines and goes directly to your blood stream), between breakfast and lunch, and another tablet between lunch and dinner.

*SAFETY ISSUES:* None.

**DHEA**

DHEA (dehyroepiandrosterone), extracted from animal glands, is the rage these days as a youth tonic. DHEA is a male hormone pumped out by the adrenal glands that has little masculinizing and much tissue-building activity. In animal studies, DHEA replacement fights obesity, protects against diabetes, sharpens memory, and wards off infectious diseases. It is also thought to buffer the effects of stress hormones and prevent age-related diseases. Low DHEA has been linked to breast cancer, obesity, high cholesterol, hypertension, heart disease, and low sex drive.

Even under normal circumstances, DHEA levels decline by as much as 75 percent between early adulthood and old age. Although no long-term studies have yet provided solid information on its benefits and side effects, short-term studies indicate that 50 mg daily for six months produced "a remarkable increase" in physical and psychological well-being, deeper sleep, increased libido, and an improved ability to handle stress. Many doctors recommend DHEA to older people for maintaining skin tone, bone density, and muscle mass.

*SAFETY ISSUES:* Though DHEA has been in use in Europe for many years as an antiobesity and anti-aging measure, some scientists warn that high doses can lead to liver damage and excessive testosterone levels. No one under thirty should take DHEA—unless under special circumstances—and no one should exceed a daily DHEA dose of 50 mg. Those who are sensitive to DHEA (the appearance of acne is a good warning that you've exceeded your limit) may be able to circumvent that sensitivity by taking its precursor, pregnenolone. Pregnenolone supplements can boost your DHEA levels, so that you receive its benefits without taking too high a dose.

Although both these supplements are available without a prescription, DHEA is a powerful hormone. You need to get your blood levels of this hormone checked before taking it, and you must continue monitoring your blood levels at regular intervals in order to determine your optimum dosage. Dosage is usually increased in gradual increments of 5 mg.

### Exercise

Virtually any exercise that includes aerobic and strengthening elements is key to maintaining sexual function as we age. Many men's problems are simply due to lack of exercise and being overweight. Chapter 4 gives you valuable information on Western and Eastern exercises. Studies show that weight lifting increases production of myofibrillar protein in aging men, strengthening their overall musculature and enhancing the contraction response that underlies all movement (including orgasms). Strong, supple muscles are essential to a healthy sex life and to enjoying powerful orgasms. Eastern exercises, including yoga postures and such Taoist exercises as the Deer, are specifically designed to protect and enhance sexual function throughout your life.

### Regular Acupuncture and/or Acupressure Treatments

Acupuncture increases circulation of blood, lymph, and energy, and is also highly effective in treating erectile dysfunction, whether the underlying cause is physical or emotional.

Self-treat the acupressure points described in chapters 4 and 11 to increase sexual potency.

### Mind Power

Chapter 5 shows you how to use visualization and imagination to enhance your sexuality and ensure good health and sexual vigor throughout your life.

## Aging and Women

Aging men are more concerned about being able to perform, while aging women are primarily worried about their appearance. Their primary fear is that men won't be excited by their bodies.

Older women seldom have physical problems that prevent orgasm. If you are having this difficulty, your only obstacle could be that you are denying yourself sexual pleasure because of your misconceptions and fears. Mature bodies don't respond as rapidly or automatically, so all you and your partner may need is to "work" together a little longer at foreplay and intercourse. If only all work was as pleasurable! In fact, this experience can bring you closer together and make your lovemaking more exciting and fulfilling.

## FEMALE MENOPAUSE AND SEXUAL DESIRE

The same sexual rule is as true for aging women as it is for aging men: Use it or lose it! Female menopause—the natural conclusion of menstruation that generally takes place in women between the ages of forty-five and fifty-five—is inevitable. But some women mistakenly equate menopause with the end of female sexual desire and activity. Not true! Let's examine the facts.

A woman officially enters menopause after she has not had a period for one year. The two or more years before menopause are referred to as "perimenopause."

The severity of symptoms among menopausal women varies greatly. About 70 to 85 percent experience some symptoms, including hot flashes, night sweats, and vaginal dryness due to lowered estrogen levels. Other side effects thought to be associated with menopause include increased risk of osteoporosis (loss of bone density), heart disease, and high cholesterol. These symptoms and hormone shifts can play havoc on a woman's sense of well-being and esteem, and some of the changes caused by menopause can impact on her sexuality.

When estrogen levels plummet, the flow of blood to the vagina can also lower, resulting in a decreased ability to feel pleasure. Some women do lose the desire for sex, but that is only partially due to hormonal changes and other symptoms such as vaginal dryness. All these conditions can be corrected. Once again, negative attitudes about aging and being attractive to a sexual partner are more likely reasons for loss of libido. A woman who has regular sex with an understanding partner is more likely to remain sexually responsive than one who doesn't.

All postmenopausal changes in sexual response are not necessarily negative. Many women get through "the change of life" with few actual changes and minimal discomfort, and they find that sex is better than ever. Women who suffered through heavy, painful, or prolonged menstrual periods often feel liberated. In fact, some postmenopausal women report greater interest in sex, as well as greater satisfaction, because they no longer fear becoming pregnant and because virtually all the discomforts associated with menopause are treatable.

In many other world cultures, including those of the East, menopause is regarded as a positive stepping-stone in a woman's life, one that marks entry into a new status as a source of wisdom and a figure of great respect.

As with everything else in life, who you were before menopause suggests a great deal about how you'll be after menopause. Among the other factors that predict how you'll navigate this life passage are your attitudes about aging, the quality of your health, and your self-esteem.

If you never enjoyed sex, menopause is a good excuse to close up shop altogether. If you've always loved to make love, at the most, you will be a bit more discriminating because raging hormones are no longer clouding your choice of partners.

## THE QUESTION OF HORMONE REPLACEMENT THERAPY (HRT)

Whether or not women should take estrogen and other hormone supplements (hormone replacement therapy, or HRT) is a subject of much debate. Advocates cite benefits to heart, bones, elimination of menopausal symptoms like hot flashes, and better sexual function. Detractors cite studies that find an increased risk of breast, ovary, and uterine cancers associated with HRT. The controversy is fierce, with some in the middle opining that cancer risk is diminished when progestin is added to the estrogen.

Of course, you must make your own choice after evaluating the research and, in consultation with your doctor, based on your individual condition and needs.

Many women choose HRT to prevent bone density loss. But estrogen alone cannot prevent osteoporosis. Studies find that along with the hormone, a woman must take calcium-magnesium supplements and practice weight-bearing exercises at least three times a week.

Some doctors are also prescribing estrogen-testosterone supplementation for postmenopausal women who complain of lack of libido. Men with the same problem are also sometimes prescribed testosterone supplements.

Warning: If you have been on HRT and wish to switch to more natural supplementation, go off your medication slowly to avoid rebound hot flashes and other symptoms, which could become worse than what you experienced before you started HRT. Begin natural replacements while weaning yourself off your artificial hormones. Always consult your doctor for specific instructions.

Once you are on the alternative route, re-evaluate your situation annually. This includes having a doctor assess your risk of heart disease and taking bone density tests.

### *Natural Progesterone Creams*

Many women have opted for applying female hormones topically through such natural products as ProGest cream, which contains progesterone, to stimulate your body's own production of hormones. ProGest is made by extracting hormonelike properties from the wild yam root that grows along North America's east coast. It produces an estrogenlike effect that relieves the symptoms of perimenopause and menopause. Ingesting the root in any other form is ineffective, as the liver filters out 99 percent of its active ingredients. Women apply a teaspoon of the cream twice a day either to the inside of the thighs, the underside of the arms, or the breasts.

This alternative is particularly helpful to perimenopausal women and seems to pose less risk of side effects than taking hormones orally.

ProGest is available over the counter. Some women even use ProGest on their faces to help reduce wrinkling. Only do this if your skin is unbroken.

Beware of other so-called "natural" estrogen and progesterone replacements. Many advertise wild yam extract content but may actually contain synthetic pharmaceutical estrogen and progesterone—in concentrations that exempt them from FDA labeling requirements.

## HOW TO REMAIN HEALTHY AND SEXUALLY TURNED ON AFTER MENOPAUSE

Almost all the guidelines for older men regarding diet, exercise, herbs, and supplements, apply to older women. Here are additional tips that are key to ensuring a healthy, happy sex life in a woman's mature years.

Follow all the advice regarding nutrition given in chapter 1. If you are smoking, quit. If you are drinking excessive amounts of alcohol and/or caffeine, cut down. Keep dietary intake of fat at or below 30 percent of your total daily calories. Eat plenty of whole grains, vegetables, and fruit and stick to healthy fats.

Our fruits, vegetables, and grains are grown in soil that lacks trace minerals (also important to immune system function, which declines as we age), and conventional dairy products come from cows that graze on pesticide-ridden grass and are pumped full of antibiotics. Since pesticides are full of harmful pseudo-estrogens that bind to your body's estrogen-receptor site where they can cause damage, it's a good idea to switch to organic food. Some experts even believe that pesticides are among the main culprits in breast cancer.

Make sure that you are eating enough foods that are high in vitamins E, A, C, B complex (folic acid is especially important), and bioflavonoids, as well as the minerals phosphorus, calcium, magnesium, iron, and zinc. See the lists in chapter 1.

In addition, certain foods have been found to exert powerfully beneficial effects on menopausal women:

### *Soybean Products*

Natural health-care providers and researchers are excited about soybeans and other foods that contain high amounts of plant hormones call phytoestrogens. Phytoestrogens also bind to the body's estrogen-receptor sites. But they mimic the effect of "good" estrogen in the body and increase the body's levels of this hormone. This is why a diet rich in soybeans eases menopausal symptoms.

Australian studies showed that consumption of 45 mg of soy flour for twelve weeks contributed to a 40 percent drop in the occurrence of hot flashes, compared to a 60 percent drop in the number of hot flashes after three months on HRT.

In Japan, where the national diet includes frequent servings of soybeans and soy products, there are so few incidences of hot flashes that they don't even have a name for them. In fact, only about 10 percent of Japanese women complain of hot flashes, while 60 percent of American postmenopausal women report experiencing hot flashes. Japanese postmenopausal women also experience a lower incidence of heart disease and hip fractures. Phytoestrogens are also thought to protect against breast cancer and heart attacks and to build extra bone mass. In addition, studies have found that phytoestrogens are risk-free.

Most experts recommend that women approaching fifty should reduce their intake of meat and chicken and increase their soy protein intake. You can easily consume two cups of soy products a day, in the form of beans, tofu, tempeh, or soy milk. (To lower cholesterol, at least two or three cups of soy products are recommended daily.)

Soybean products such as tofu, soy milk, and miso are not the only foods that contain significant levels of phytoestrogens. Green peas, green beans, dried beans, split peas, lentils, oats, rice, wheat, and sesame seeds are also rich in this plant estrogen.

### *Cruciferous Veggies*

Another class of foods that is particularly helpful in the middle years are cruciferous vegetables—broccoli, cauliflower, kale, brussels sprouts, turnips, rutabaga, and cabbage. These contain a powerful phytochemical called indole-3-carbinol (IC3) that has cancer-fighting properties, especially against breast cancer that may be caused by an excess amount of artificial estrogen.

### *Flaxseed Oil*

Regular doses of flaxseed oil, a golden-colored oil that tastes like butter, also produces an estrogenlike effect on the body. Cooking destroys the oil's benefits, so add it after cooking. Your daily intake of flaxseed oil should total one to two tablespoons. See chapter 1 for more specific recommendations.

### *Acidophilus*

Postmenopausal women are also more susceptible to yeast infections, because lack of estrogen leaves the vaginal wall drier and thinner, and its pH changes from acid to alkaline—all ideal conditions for yeast overgrowth. Keep your intestinal tract and vagina colonized with helpful bacteria by consuming yogurt daily or by taking an acidophilus supplement. If you are allergic to dairy products, nondairy acidophilus supplements are available. If you suffer from chronic yeast infections, avoid acidophilus in any form until you can reduce the yeast overgrowth by taking citrus seed extract, caprylic acid, or Tanalbit (which combines natural vitamins with zinc). When the yeast infections have abated, you can resume acidophilus intake to restore microbe balance in your system. Follow other directions for avoiding yeast infections given in chapter 1.

### *Herbal Menopause Remedies*

Certain herbs are especially helpful to aging women and can balance hormone levels well enough to preclude the use of HRT.

The Chinese herbal tradition is considered most effective for countering the effects of aging, and in particular the symptoms of menopause and low libido. These ancient formulations usually include ginseng and dong quai, which boost sex organ and gland function in aging women and exert a toning action overall. While both herbs are widely available as single remedies, in capsule and fluid extract forms, the ideal approach would be to consult an expert in Chinese herbology who can prescribe a formula especially for you.

Western herbalists recommend the above herbs, as well as others. Depending on your overall condition and the pattern and severity of your symptoms, you can take any of the following herbs, either alone or in compound remedies. The most commonly used herbs for the treatment of menopause are angelica (aka dong quai), licorice root (*Glycyrrhiza glabra*), black cohosh (*Cimicifuga racemosa*), sarsparilla root (*Smilex officinalis*), and ginseng.

#### BLACK COHOSH (CIMICIFUGA RACEMOSA)

Black cohosh is considered to be “estriol-like” in activity. Estriol is a weak form of estrogen made by our bodies that helps strengthen and thicken the vaginal lining. Clinical studies have shown that black cohosh decreases the incidence of depression, vaginal dryness, and hot flashes without any known side effects. Daily use of black cohosh extracts can provide relief from menopausal symptoms within a few months. The standardized extract called Remifemin, made by Enzymatic Therapy, is one of the finest and in clinical trials compares favorably with HRT.

Black cohosh should be taken along with panax ginseng. Follow dose instructions on bottle label.

### Borage (Borago Officinalis)

Borage is a great toner for the adrenals, which, in turn, helps to maintain sexual function. Borage oil, taken in capsules, pills, or as part of a compound supplement, is one of the most effective and widely prescribed treatments for the symptoms of menopause.

Follow dose instructions on the bottle label for borage oil. You can also make a tea, using either one teaspoon of dried flowers or two to three teaspoons of dried leaves steeped in half a cup of hot water. Do not use for over a month at a time.

### Dong Quai (Angelica)

Also known as the female hormone herb or the female ginseng, dong quai is actually one of at least ten species of angelica and is a longtime staple in Chinese herbal formulas that is becoming increasingly popular here in the West. It is particularly effective in countering the troubling symptoms that often accompany menopause and is often prescribed in conjunction with chaste berry for this purpose.

Standard dose is three times daily of one teaspoon of the fluid extract. In other forms, follow the dosage instructions on the bottle label. Though dong quai is generally considered safe, some of its chemical components can interact with sunlight and cause a rash or severe sunburn.

### FEVERFEW (TANACETUM PARTHENIUM)

Feverfew is an effective remedy for menopause-related migraines, as well as for other symptoms of menopause.

*DOSE:* Feverfew is available in loose, dried form, tea bags, capsules, and tinctures. However, for any preparation to be effective, it must contain about .25 to .5 mg of parthenolide, feverfew's active ingredient. So, the best form of this herb is standardized tablets or capsules that contain a consistent amount of its active principles. Take two a day, but do not use for over four to six weeks at a time or you can develop cold sores, fever blisters, or a skin rash.

### LICORICE ROOT (GLYCYRRHIZA GLABRA)

The roots of licorice contain health-enhancing phytoestrogens that, like soy products, bind to estrogen sites and help balance hormones, increase estrogen metabolism, and relieve menopausal symptoms. Licorice is also known as "the great harmonizer" in Chinese medicine, because this tasty root sweetens many tonic formulas. The root is available in whole form in health food stores and Asian herbal stores. It is also widely available in tea, capsule, and tincture form. The dose is based on the content level of its active ingredients, particularly glycyrrhizin. Take one to two capsules a day. Avoid if you have high blood pressure.

### GINSENG, PANAX AND SIBERIAN

Panax ginseng (aka Korean or Chinese ginseng) is an all-over toner, strengthener, and stimulator that supports the sex organs and glands and can be taken indefinitely. Panax ginseng works by preserving the health of female reproductive tissues during menopause or following a hysterectomy, by stimulating the body's own production of estrogen. A daily regime of panax ginseng can be enough to prevent the atrophic vaginal changes associated with menopause symptoms. Since panax ginseng is an adaptogen, you can usually take it as long as you want.

Siberian ginseng also has a general toning action that is helpful to menopausal women, but it is more effective in clearing the mind (short-term memory loss is another common accompaniment to menopause) than in supporting sex organ gland function.

*DOSE:* This depends on the content of ginsenoside, the active ingredient in panax ginseng. Take one capsule per day that contains at least .5 percent ginsenoside. Menopausal women often benefit from taking ginseng in conjunction with black cohosh.

### Saw Palmetto (Serenoa Repens)

Though this herb is usually prescribed for men, especially aging men at risk for prostatitis, it can also benefit menopausal women with thinning vaginal walls. Take one 80 to 200 mg capsule standardized to give 85 to 95 percent of fatty acid sterols after each meal. The key is standardization. The lower dose is tonic; the higher dose is corrective.

### Herbal Teas

Instead of coffee or caffeinated tea, you can substitute teas made from any of the above herbs, as well as anise, chaste berry, red clover, sarsaparilla, and fennel. Medical studies on their efficacy have only gotten underway, but anecdotal evidence suggests that any of these teas can help you feel stronger, more energetic, and reduce menopausal symptoms. Of course, all herbs are more potent in standardized extract form. Try a tea first, to see if that form is strong enough for you.

*DOSE:* Drink one to three cups a day.

*SAFETY ISSUES:* Since these herbs can exert powerful effects on blood pressure and heart rhythm—especially in fluid extract form—if you have any chronic health problems, you should consult your doctor before taking them.

If your libido is low, try either kava kava, muira puama, or yohimbe half an hour before sex, following the instructions given in chapter 10.

You can also take compound sex tonics daily. Try the Chinese Female-Strengthening Tonic (one to two tablespoons daily), Fennel-Licorice Sex Tonic (two tablespoons, twice a day), or Chinese Chicken Soup for Women (drink freely). Follow the recipes for these tonics given in chapter 2.

### *Take Supplements*

All the supplements recommended in chapter 3 will help to preserve health and act as rejuvenators for menopausal women. Since your supply of certain essential vitamins, minerals, and other body chemicals lowers with age, along with your body's ability to metabolize them, you need to take certain supplements. The smartest idea is to visit your health-care provider and request to have your vitamin and mineral blood levels taken. Then take whatever supplements you need to make up for any deficits.

The following supplements are particularly helpful to the menopausal woman:

*VITAMIN E:* between 800 and 1,000 I.U.s a day is helpful against vaginal atrophy and dryness. Some doctors recommend topical applications of vitamin E oil to vaginal tissues, but that can provoke an allergic response. Plus, if the E is from a bottle instead of a fresh capsule, it can be easily contaminated by germs on your hands, no matter how clean you may think they are.

*BORON:* 6 mg three times a day helps counter symptoms of female menopause.

*FOLIC ACID:* 20 mg three times a day is also extremely effective in relieving menopausal symptoms.

*ZINC:* 60 mg a day helps the thymus gland continue to manufacture hormones called thymosins, which, in turn, stimulate production of neurotransmitters and sex hormones.

*CALCIUM:* 1,000 to 1,500 mg a day along with half that amount of magnesium is essential to maintain bone density and health. Follow the recommendations given above in the section on aging men and supplements regarding vitamin D and sunshine to help metabolize calcium and magnesium.

*BEE POLLEN:* If you use bee pollen, take only the granular form. Safeguard yourself against allergic reactions by starting off with only one grain per meal. Increase by one grain per meal each day, until you reach a total dose level of one teaspoon per day.

*MELATONIN:* See the section above regarding supplements for aging men. The same recommendations hold true for aging women.

DHEA: See the section above regarding supplements for aging men. The same recommendations hold true for aging women.

### *Exercise*

Get regular exercise, including aerobic exercise, stretching and exercise involving weights. Weight-bearing exercises not only help maintain bone density in postmenopausal women, they boost muscle proteins called myofibrillar proteins in both sexes.

Yoga gives you a youthful suppleness and flexibility. It also helps prevent "dowager's hump," a curvature in the upper back seen in many aging women, and ensures that your breathing remains deep and balanced. All these are essentials for everlasting youth and sexual vitality.

Kegeling and Taoist exercises are among the greatest gifts you can give yourself. They are tremendously rejuvenating because they keep your love muscles, as well as your entire body, toned, flexible, and operating smoothly. They will also ensure your continuing capacity for sexual pleasure.

Involve your partner in exercising, as in all your efforts to create a healthier lifestyle. You will both benefit from the changes.

### *Acupressure Treatments*

The balancing and restorative effects of acupressure are literally at your fingertips. If you stimulate certain points listed in chapter 4, you can increase your sexual energy any time, at your convenience and absolutely free. Acupressure is less powerful than acupuncture, but you can apply it any time you desire.

## SPECIAL POINTS FOR MENOPAUSE SYMPTOMS

Hot flashes and other abrupt shifts in body temperature are due to the sudden decrease of estrogen levels. Estrogen is regulated by the pituitary gland, which is also in charge of body temperature. Use the following acupressure points one to four times a day to balance your pituitary and other endocrine glands, stabilize blood pressure, and reduce flushing. As you apply pressure to the following points, focus your mind on the benefits implied by their colorfully descriptive names.

*Bubbling Springs*

Location: At the ball of the foot, between the two pads.
Benefits: Relieves hot flashes, fainting, convulsions.

*Elegant Mansion*

Location: In the hollow below the collarbone, next to the breastbone.
Benefits: Relieves hot flashes, depression, breathing difficulties.

*Joining the Valley*

Location: In the webbing between the thumb and index finger, at the highest spot of the muscle when the thumb and index finger are brought together.
Benefits: Relieves hot flashes.

*Gates of Consciousness*

Location: Below the base of the skull, in the hollows two to three inches apart, depending on the size of the head.
Benefits: Relieves hot flashes and headaches, dizziness, irritability.

*Sea of Tranquility*

Location: On the center of the breastbone, three thumb-widths up from the base of the bone.
Benefits: Relieves hot flashes, nervousness, anxiety, insomnia, depression, and emotional distress.

*Third Eye Point*

Location: Directly between the eyebrows, in the indentation where the bridge of the nose meets the forehead.

Benefits: Helps the endocrine system, especially the pituitary gland, relieves hot flashes and headaches.

### *One Hundred Meeting Point*

Location: On the crown of the head in an indentation or "soft spot" between the cranial bones. To find the point, follow the line from the back of the ears to the top of the head.

Benefits: Improves mental concentration and memory, relieves headaches and hot flashes.

Regular massage is also helpful. Massage keeps you in touch with your sensuality, calms frazzled nerves, relieves muscular tensions, and helps your body cleanse itself of toxins and increase blood and lymph circulation.

### *Stay Sexually Active*

Regular sexual arousal stimulates hormone production and minimizes vaginal changes that sometimes occur with menopause. Studies indicate that making love at least once a week raises levels of estrogen, helping to maintain elasticity in vaginal tissue. Menopause can cause vaginal tissues to become more sensitive to irritation and infection, and intercourse may become uncomfortable. A water-based lubricant should alleviate that problem. In addition, any type of sexual activity, including masturbation, helps maintain and improve vaginal lubrication. On the other hand, if you go too long without sexual stimulation, when you finally do make love or masturbate, you will probably encounter problems with vaginal thinning, dryness, or inability to lubricate. If that sexual experience is painful or otherwise unpleasant, you may make the mistake of giving up on sex altogether.

Consult chapters 6, 8, and 9 for ways in which to restore fun, passion, and excitement to your love life. Here's a simple tip: Pretend that you and your partner are young and dating again; relive those exciting days of petting. Also, tantric and Taoist lovemaking are ideally suited for the older couple. See chapter 8 for complete descriptions and instructions.

Be patient. You may no longer have a hair-trigger response to sexual stimulation, but you can become just as aroused as before.

And it's more fun if you take your time. Again, if you find yourself drier than before menopause, use a water-based lubricant.

Create and practice visualizations to restore your self-image as a sexual being. See chapter 5 for instructions and suggestions for scenarios.

Be open with friends and anyone who can share valuable information about menopause. In many circles of our culture, menopause is still considered a taboo topic and even somewhat of an embarassment. Women can experience menopause as a wound to their femininity. Some become depressed, project their negative feelings onto their partners, and even create situations that lead to divorce.

Armed with these natural remedies and positive attitudes, menopause can mark the passage into your mature, wise woman years, when experience brings you the gift of self-acceptance and a clearer, more accurate view on life.

## A FINAL WORD . . .

If you approach aging with fear and dread, frantically searching for magic formulas to keep you young and sexually appealing, you will only increase the power of these forces that age you before your time. The guidance and recommendations given in this chapter and in all the previous chapters of this book will give you long life, good health, and youthful attractiveness. They are also your best insurance against losing sexual vigor and enjoyment.

These contentions are supported by Western science. Studies consistently find that sex is good for you at any age. It has been proven that touch, sexual or otherwise, boosts immune function, and that the more sexually satisfied you are, the less likely you are to be depressed. Even the onset of senility is proven to be directly related to loss of sexuality.

Most important, the longer you remain sexually active, the less likely you are to experience a weakening of your bodily functions and a loss of your physical and mental vitality. Follow the advice presented in this book, and you will find that you can retard the actual process and enjoy great sex at any age.

Life-long sexual passion and youthful vitality can become your reality. Now that you have all the necessary information, making it happen is up to you.

# Resource Guide


BOOKS ON NATURAL HEALING AND SEX, GENERAL

Atkins, Robert C. *Dr. Atkins Health Revolution: How Complementary Medicine Can Extend Your Life* (Bantam, 1990).

Bechtel, Stefan. *The Practical Encyclopedia of Sex and Health: From Aphrodisiacs and Hormones to Potency, Stress, Vasectomy and Yeast Infections* (Rodale Press, 1993).

Brody, Jane. *Jane Brody's Guide to Personal Health* (Avon Books, 1982).

DeMoya, Armando and Dorothy, and Lewis, Martha E. and Howard R. *Sex and Health: A Practical Guide to Sexual Medicine* (Stein and Day, 1983).

Flatto, Edwin. *Super Potency at Any Age* (Instant Improvement, Inc., 1991).

Kordel, Lelord. *Natural Folk Remedies* (Putnam, 1974).

Scott, Julian and Susan. *Natural Medicine for Women* (Gaia Books, 1991).

BOOKS ON DIET

Phillips, David A. *Guidebook to Nutritional Factors in Foods* (Woodbridge Press, 1979).

Salaman, Maureen with James F. Scheer. *Foods That Heal* (Statford, 1989).

Walker, Joan and Morton. *Sexual Nutrition: The Lover's Diet* (Zebra, 1983).

Walker, Morton. *Sexual Nutrition: How to Nutritionally Improve, Enhance, and Stimulate Your Sexual Appetite* (Avery, 1994).

Yetiv, Jack Z. *Popular Nutritional Practices: Sense and Nonsense* (Dell, 1988).

For cookbooks with imaginative recipes that use the soy bean:

Rombauer, Irma. *The Joy of Cooking* (Simon & Schuster, 1997).

Shandler, Nina. *Estrogen: The Natural Way* (Villard, 1997).

## BOOKS ON HERBAL REMEDIES

Elias, Jason and Masline, Shelagh Ryan. *The A to Z Guide to Healing Herbal Remedies* (Dell, 1995).

Fratkin, Jake. *Chinese Herbal Patent Formulas: A Practical Guide* (Shya, 1991).

Kloss, Jethro. *Back to Eden* (Woodbridge Press, 1983).

Lucas, Richard. *Common & Uncommon Uses of Herbs for Healthier Living* (Arc, 1969).

Lust, John. *The Herb Book* (Bantam, 1980).

Mitton, Mervyn. *Herbal Remedies: Sexual Remedies* (Foulsham, 1992).

Murray, Michael T. *The Healing Power of Herbs: The Enlightened Person's Guide to the Wonders of Medicinal Plants* (Prima, 1995).

Oumano, Elena. *A Handbook of Natural Folk Remedies* (Avon, 1997).

Parvati, Jeannine. *Hygeia: A Woman's Herbal* (Freestone Collective, 1978).

Rose, Jeanne. *Herbs & Things: Jeanne Rose's Herbal* (Workman, 1972).

Shelagh, Ryan Masline and Close, Barbara. *The A–Z Guide to Healing with Essential Oils* (Dell, 1997).

Tierra, Michael. *The Way of Herbs* (Washington Square Press, 1983).

Weed, Susun S. *The Wise Woman Herbal: Childbearing Years* (Ash Tree, 1986).

Worwood, Valerie Ann. *The Complete Book of Essential Oils & Aromatherapy* (New World Library, 1991).

## BOOKS ON SUPPLEMENTS

DeCava, Judith A. *The Real Truth about Vitamins and Antioxidants* (Brentwood Academic Press, 1996).

Mindell, Earl. *Earl Mindell's Vitamin Bible* (Warner, 1979).

## BOOKS ON ACUPRESSURE AND ACUPUNCTURE

Chan, Pedro. *Finger Acupressure* (Ballantine, 1975).

Gach, Michael Reed. *Acupressure's Potent Points: A Guide to Self-Care for Common Ailments* (Bantam, 1990).

Ohashi, Wataru. *Do-It-Yourself Shiatsu* (Dutton, 1976).

Teeguarden, Iona Marsaa. *Acupressure Way of Health: Jin Shin Do* (Japan, 1978).

## BOOKS ON EASTERN LOVEMAKING PHILOSOPHIES AND PRACTICES

Most books that interpret Eastern sexual philosophies for modern Western lovers are not very accessible to the average couple who may not be interested in the spiritual theories. The following titles do, however, expand on many points included in this book's discussion.

Anand, Margo. *The Art of Sexual Ecstasy: The Path of Sacred Sexuality for Western Lovers* (Tarcher, 1989).
Blofeld, John. *The Tantric Mysticism of Tibet* (Dutton, 1970).
Chang, Stephen T. with Miller, Richard C. *The Book of Internal Exercises* (Strawberry Hill Press, 1980).
Chang, Stephen T. *The Great Tao* (Tao Publishing, 1987).
Chia, Mantak and Maneewan, and Winn, Michael. *Taoist Secrets of Love: Cultivating Male Sexual Energy* (Aurora Press, 1984).
Chia, Mantak and Maneewan. *Healing Love Through the Tao: Cultivating Female Sexual Energy* (Healing Tao Books, 1986).
Garrison, Omar. *Tantra: The Yoga of Sex* (Causeway, 1964).
Haich, Elisabeth. *Sexual Energy and Yoga* (Asi, 1972).
Kushi, Michio. *The Gentle Art of Making Love: Macrobiotics in Love and Sexuality* (Avery, 1990).
Masters, Jean and Robert. *Mind Games: The Guide to Inner Space* (Delta, 1972).
Oki, Mashahito. *Zen Yoga Therapy* (Japan, 1979).

In addition, many workshops and seminars across the country, particularly in California, teach the ways of Eastern sex. For information on tantric sexuality workshops, call the New York Open Center (212-219-2527) or Charles and Caroline Muir at Hawaiian Goddess (808-572-8364). For further information on Taoist exercises, contact: The Healing Tao Center, P.O. Box 1194, Huntington, NY 11743; telephone: 516-367-2701.

## BOOKS ON BODY-MIND AWARENESS

Bry, Adelaide with Bair, Marjorie. *Visualization: Directing the Movie of Your Mind* (Barnes & Noble, 1972).
DeMille, Richard. *Put Your Mother on the Ceiling: Children's Imagination Games* (Penguin, 1973).
Lowen, Alexander. *Love and Orgasm: A Revolutionary View of the Role of Love in Sex* (Signet, 1967).
Lowen, Alexander. *The Betrayal of the Body* (Collier, 1967).
Lubetkin, Barry and Oumano, Elena. *Bailing Out: The Healthy Way to Get Out of a Bad Relationship and Survive* (Prentice Hall Press, 1991).
Mumford, Susan. *The Complete Guide to Massage* (Plume, 1996).
Pelletier, Kenneth R. *Mind As Healer, Mind As Slayer: A Holistic Approach to Preventing Stress Disorder* (Delta, 1977).

Purvis, Kenneth. *The Male Sexual Machine: An Owner's Manual* (St. Martin's Press, 1992).
Reich, Wilhelm. *The Function of the Orgasm* (Bantam, 1961).
Reuben, David. *How to Get More Out of Sex* (Bantam, 1974).
Sanford, John A. *Between People: Communicating One-to-One* (Paulist Press, 1982).
Selye, Hans. *Stress Without Distress* (Signet, 1974).

## MAIL ORDER COMPANIES

For organic foods, supplements and herbal remedies:

Lifethyme store
212-420-9099
Ask for David I. F. Miller, biochemist/nutritional consultant

Whole Foods store
212-982-1000/Fax: 212-982-0186

Hickey Chemists, Ltd. (supplements, herbs, homeopathic remedies)
800-724-5566

L & H Vitamins
800-221-1152

Vitamin Direct
800-468-4027

Freeda Vitamins
800-777-3737

Needs
800-634-1380

Mother's Choice
888-HERB-MOM

AmeriHerb, Inc.
800-267-6141

A Catalogue of Herbal Delights
800-879-3337

Abundant Life Herbal Supply
510-939-7857

Aromystique
888-722-1244
on-line: www.aromystique.com

Aromatherapy
800-610-3674

Vitamin Trader
800-334-9300

Pinetree Vitamins
on-line: www.netresultz.com/pinetree
E-mail: pinetree@netresultz.com

Phillips Nutritionals
800-582-8461

Vitamin Discount Connection
888-848-2110

The Vitamin Zone
800-583-1187
on-line: www.TheVitaminZone.com

The Vitamin Shoppe
800-223-1216

East Earth Trade Winds (for Chinese herbs)
800-258-6878

Brion Herbs (for Chinese herbs)
800-333-HERB

Chinese Herbal Tonics
913-677-0890
on-line: http://kansascityguide.com/kang_le_so

Phyto Pharmacia
800-553-2370

For organic food, natural cleansers, clothing, linens:

Harmony: Products in Harmony with the Earth
800-869-3446/Fax: 800-456-1139

Self Care: Products for Healthy Living
800-345-3371

Natural Lifestyle Supplies
800-752-2775

The Allergy Store (one-stop shopping for nontoxic products)
800-824-7163

Decent Exposures (100 percent cotton comfort designed by women for women)
800-524-4949

Harmony (Seventh Generation)
800-869-3446

Janice's Natural Comfort Collection
800-Janices

Aveda stores, a national chain of natural body-care products, offers a range of fragrances made from natural essential oils.

## EQUIPMENT FOR TAOIST EGG AND WEIGHT-LIFTING VAGINAL EXERCISES

To order a catalog or equipment, call the International Healing Tao Centers headquarters: 800-497-1017

For an International Healing Tao Center in your area, call

212-330-7876

## REFERRAL FOR SEX COUNSELING

For a referral to a sex therapist, send a SASE to the American Association of Sex Educators, Counselors, and Therapists, P.O. Box 238, Mount Vernon, IA 52314-0238.

## RECOMMENDED MAGAZINES

Call the following numbers for subscription queries.

*Natural Health*
800-526-8440

*New Age*
800-782-7006

*Yoga Journal*
800-436-9642

*American Health for Women*
800-365-5005

*Men's Health*
800-666-2303

*Alternative Medicine Digest*
415-435-1779

*Fitness*
800-888-1181

# Index